PROTECTING MENTAL HEALTH

Dr Keith Gaynor works as a senior clinical psychologist in the Outpatient Department of St John of God Hospital, Stillorgan. He specialises in Cognitive Behavioural Therapy (CBT) treatments of anxiety and depression. Keith trained at Kings College London and University College Dublin. He has written widely in academic journals on the topic of CBT and is a regular contributor to the Irish media, including *The Tubridy Show*, *Prime Time* and *The Irish Independent*, on issues of mental health.

Protecting
MENTAL HEALTH

Dr Keith Gaynor

VERITAS

Published 2015 by Veritas Publications
7–8 Lower Abbey Street
Dublin 1, Ireland
publications@veritas.ie
www.veritas.ie

ISBN 978 1 84730 630 2

10 9 8 7 6 5 4 3 2 1

A catalogue record for this book is available from the British Library.

Designed by Heather Costello, Veritas Publications
Printed by SPRINT-print Ltd, Dublin

*Veritas books are printed on paper made from the wood pulp of managed
forests. For every tree felled, at least one tree is planted, thereby renewing
natural resources.*

Dedication

To Fiona, who is always the last kiss before wartime.

Contents

Prologue

Humans didn't survive sixty thousand years of evolution alone. We hunt in packs. We live in tribes. We raise children in communities. We are a social animal. As I write this, the All-Ireland GAA football championship is coming to a conclusion. Team, parish, county and country bind us together. Yet we work in offices and cubicles. We drive alone in cars. We shut out the world around us by wearing earphones on buses. Without any effort, it is quite easy to spend large parts of our day alone. Even when we sit together, how connected are we? It is too easy to be lonely in a crowded room. We have to make an effort to form a real connection, to have a real conversation. We have to make an effort so that each encounter has some real meaning to it. The busyness of our lives and noisiness of our world means that connections can often drift apart.

Many of us kissed someone goodbye this morning. How often does that kiss have real meaning? This, the most important person in the world to us, gets a peck on the cheek, a shout from the door, a grunt and a groan as we rush away to do something more important. Yet if we knew this was our last day, what would that kiss be like? Without doubt, it would be one hell of a thing. It would matter. I have a wonderful daydream involving thousands of people bowling their partners over with fantastic last-kiss-before-wartime goodbyes. The Romans said *carpe diem*. The Buddhists said live in the moment. This book is about how to enjoy life *that* much. It is about how to give the last kiss before wartime.

Acknowledgements

I would like to thank everyone at St John of God Hospital –
this book would not have been possible without their wisdom
and kindness; and Margaret and Cormac – everything good I
ever learned, I learned first at home.

Three Revolutions

'Hope' is the thing with feathers –
That perches in the soul –
And sings the tune without the words –
And never stops – at all –
EMILY DICKINSON

In the ten years I have been a psychologist, I have met hundreds of people in the course of my work. Many have struggled with extraordinary psychological and emotional difficulties. People have been racked with anxiety, have felt the darkest lows, have heard voices or been crippled by fear or paranoia. The truth, seldom articulated, is that most people get better. These things happen but we get through them.

The colleague in the room next to mine told me the other day that the most common sound she hears coming from my office is laughter, mine and my clients'. That might sound positive to you, but as a therapist it got me quite worried. Was I glossing over people's difficulties? Was I avoiding the hard questions and the tough emotions? I mulled it over. Ultimately, I decided I was doing something, intuitively, which is vital in therapy. I was embodying a hopeful spirit and inviting the clients to do the same. People were finding tiny glimmers of light in their situations, however challenging.

The reason we laugh in sessions is because we constantly find little shafts of brightness and, in those moments, hope is born. Not everyone laughs – and plenty of people cry – but for each person, seeking out that genuine emotion allows them to connect to that most human part of themselves. All therapy begins in hope: in the hope of feeling better, in the hope of suffering less, in the hope of enjoying life. It mightn't always be apparent. We sometimes have to work a little bit to find it but hope is always there, just beneath the surface.

Friends often ask me if being a psychologist is depressing and I can honestly say it isn't. People start from a difficult place. No one comes to a psychologist because life is wonderful. But you get to sit with people as a minor miracle happens: they become happy. I'm able to laugh because it is a joy to be with someone in those moments but also because I know even if we are not there yet, most people will get there. I know the statistics and the recovery rates and I've seen it countless times with my own eyes. It is a myth that people don't recover from mental health problems. People get better all the time. They go back to work and to their families and move on with their lives. I know this from my own family and friends. Students have a difficult couple of months in college but eventually get back on course. People return to their jobs and their lives. Couples have a difficult period in their marriage but twenty years later it seems like a blip. Therapy isn't about developing coping skills or the capacity to merely muddle through. It is about complete recovery. It is about getting to the point where you are just content.

Yet significant changes are needed if we, as a community, are to achieve good mental health. To my mind, we need to understand three things if we want to achieve good mental health. These aren't small things. In fact, if we were really to engage with them, they would be revolutionary.

1. As individuals, we need to understand *how* to be happy
2. As individuals, we need to understand how to *reduce* unhappiness
3. As a society, we need to understand *how* to create a happier country.

DENTAL AND MENTAL HEALTH

We treat our mental lives quite differently from how we treat our physical lives. How many times will you brush your teeth today? Twice? Three times? But what will you do to nurture your psychological well-being? If you are like most people, you probably won't do much. We tend to wait until there is a crisis before we start doing anything to improve our mental health but we are far more proactive when it comes to our dental health. With our teeth, we take small positive steps every day to prevent decay. We know it is too late to start brushing when we already need dentures. We treat our mental health the same way our great-grandparents treated their teeth: to be ignored until they became overwhelmingly painful.

There is an extraordinary prejudice that nearly everyone in Ireland has. We believe mental health problems are different from physical health problems. It is perfectly acceptable to take the necessary treatment for high blood pressure, a migraine or high cholesterol. But a different attitude prevails when it comes to mental health. Many still believe that to feel overwhelmed is a sign of weakness – no matter how stressful our lives – or believe that we are to blame for feeling depressed. Even with the changes in society, it is still very common for people to believe that mental health is something shameful that needs to be hidden. We see our troubles as impossible battles that we have to struggle with forever.

Although attitudes are changing, we still have a long way to go. There's nothing magical about mental health; it isn't some unknown realm where witch doctors roam. Such attitudes came from a basic lack of knowledge about how the mind works. The last thirty years have seen an explosion in the number of publications on the subject of popular psychology and the bestsellers list has been brimming with titles that relay cutting-edge discoveries to the layperson. They include Steven Pinker's explanations of how important evolution is to our psychology; Antonio Damasio's description of the neurological underpinnings of consciousness; and Daniel Kahneman's revolutionary work on the two core processes of our brain. We have a radically improved understanding of how the mind works as a result. However, I visit my friends' houses and, though they have all these books on their shelves, they haven't necessarily deployed that knowledge in their day-to-day actions. It's like reading a book about the gym – unless you put it into practice you won't get fit.

Most people I see are already in crisis and their mental health has been declining for a while. Things have gone awry: partners may have left; they may be on long-term leave from work due to illness. These crises drive people towards mental health services. But our mental health is not unlike our dental health – if we wait for the crisis, then it is much harder to fix. We understand this intuitively about the rest of the body but we are still reluctant to embrace this reality when it comes to mental health.

We need to take responsibility for our own mental well-being. We watch our diet to reduce the risk of diabetes; we manage our fitness to reduce the risk of heart disease; we quit smoking to reduce the risk of lung disease. Over the last fifty years, our attitude to physical well-being has shifted from one of crisis intervention to preventative healthcare. Mental health is only catching up.

The pattern in most people's lives over the last twenty years has been to work harder, put more demands on themselves and, as a result, become ever more stressed. Humans are excellent doers. In fact, we can be efficient from the moment we wake in the morning to the moment we fall asleep at night. But we have become terrible at just 'being': being calm, being quiet, reading books, listening to music, being in the garden, not trying, not focusing, not having a goal.

Think of the hours of your week. What percentage of those hours allow for happiness? What hours allow for calm? For how many hours do you get to be you? We all have responsibilities and we cannot be unoccupied all the time, but is there any possibility that the ratio of work to calm has been compromised? Happiness matters and if we don't emphasise it in our lives, it disappears. It won't turn up by accident. We have to seek it out.

The first three chapters of this book look at the evidence for what makes us happy. Much of it is hardly surprising but it is in danger of slipping away, and if we value our own happiness we have to fight to include it in our lives.

HOW NOT TO BE UNHAPPY

I work in a clinic for anxiety disorders and depression. At the moment, using a specialist cognitive behavioural therapy (CBT) approach we have an average recovery rate for those in therapy of 80 per cent. Those are people who are not just managing, not just coping or getting by, but who are as content and active as anyone else in the population. This section seeks to address the mechanics of psychological difficulties such as depression, anxiety, worry and emotional dysregulation so that we can prevent them or respond to them more quickly and effectively.

One of the privileges of being a psychologist is that patients come to talk about their lives. I've learned something amazing from those experiences. It is really hard to lose your job, break your leg, be bullied in work, or have deadlines that are impossible to meet. It is very difficult to be the mother of a newborn or be a mother of a toddler *and* a newborn; it's difficult to be old in Ireland or be young in Ireland. It can be difficult to simple 'be'. Any of these situations can make us stressed and unhappy. Yet there are lots of quick, effective treatments that will help you with those stresses but we have to seek them out and we have to use them. The pharmacist doesn't ring round the house on spec to see if you have a cold. We have to approach them.

The process and mechanics of unhappiness are specific and need to be challenged in a systematic way. Unhappiness is not just the absence of happiness. We have to understand and challenge the processes that maintain unhappiness. Thankfully, we are much further down the road of understanding these mechanics than we were thirty years ago.

The simple fact is that if people have access to evidence-based treatments, the treatments work. The major problem in mental health today isn't that there aren't treatments that work. It is that people either don't have access to them or they don't receive treatment quickly enough.

There's nothing magical about interacting with a psychologist. It is good, solid treatment that could have been availed of months or years before. In our clinic, we offer evidence-based treatment *early* in the process. And when you do it in that order, it works.

Two factors need to be in place for therapy to work:
‣ positive interaction with a stranger who is present with you through a difficult time
‣ strong evidence-based techniques that are proven to work.

This section is designed to help people address common psychological difficulties and the evidence is that this approach works for lots of people, especially if they can use the techniques before a crisis happens. We all need to be and can be our own therapist. This book lays out a series of principles that have a strong scientific backing and decades of on-the-ground practice. It is what we do in the clinic every day. None of it is revolutionary. The key is to do it. A push-up is a simple exercise but if you repeat it, it will make you strong. People often buy dozens of books on improving mental health. They *all* work if *you* work them and it is the same for this one. This is about how people can use the best psychological techniques in their own lives in an uncomplicated but very effective manner.

The middle section of this book focuses on four of the most common psychological difficulties that people face: **anxiety,**

depression, worry and **emotional dysregulation.** These can affect anyone and, for some people, can be so severe they are overwhelming. This is generally what people call a mental illness. However, we don't have to wait until it becomes an illness to deal with. We can act much earlier than that.

In this book I examine three core areas: *thoughts, emotions* and *behaviours.* They can feed into each other and create a vicious cycle that's very difficult to escape. They distort what we think, they alter what we do and they change how we feel about ourselves and the world around us. Often our natural reaction to these feelings doesn't alleviate them. In fact, we maintain them and make them worse. These are traps that so many of us fall into.

Everyone has experienced anxiety in their lives. It is an extraordinarily physical sensation that runs through every cell in the body. It is normal but it feels awful. More than anything we want to avoid it. But the paradox is that the more we avoid it, the more it increases. In order to overcome anxiety, we have to approach it slowly. If we don't understand this about our body, we will never be able to manage our anxiety.

Depression is a word we use to cover a whole spectrum of experiences. It includes low mood, low motivation, negative thoughts, physical exhaustion. It makes us reluctant to engage in our normal life, but the less we do the worse we feel. If we don't understand this about our body – that we are cavemen who need a certain level of activity – then we can never get past these feelings.

We all have important decisions to make and stressful situations to overcome in our lives. They make us worry. The paradox is that the more we put off making the decisions, the more anxious we feel. Certain decisions become so important that we can feel paralysed by them. If we don't understand the importance of balancing reflection and decision-making, it is easy to get caught up in that cycle again and again.

There is nothing shameful in becoming trapped by these paradoxes, but they are counterintuitive. You would naturally think that if you avoid anxiety you will feel better but it just doesn't hold true. There is nothing unusual in experiencing such distress. In fact, it is the most natural reaction in unpleasant situations. Everyone will experience anxiety to a certain extent and one in three people will experience it to such an extent that the problem overtakes their lives. It is not strange, not stigmatising, not unique, but a normal reaction to stressful situations that can create mental health problems. These problems can be solved by talking about them, reading books about them, hearing lectures about them, putting in some positive behavioural structures to sort them out and, if need be, seeing a psychologist or a psychiatrist to talk about them.

What I endeavour to do in the middle chapters is outline what advice and support a psychologist would provide in the first couple of sessions of therapy. These are exactly the subjects I talk to people about every day. They can seem impossible. How can you ask someone who is depressed to be motivated? How can you ask someone who is anxious not to worry? But therapy is full of these paradoxes and that is exactly what we ask people to do. The person with no motivation is asked to find some. The person overwhelmed by fear is asked to move closer to it. We ask the person to do the smallest thing that they are able to do and then to move one inch further than that.

The extraordinary, life-fulfilling, hope-giving, miracle of it all is that it works. It works in clinics; it works in scientific trials; it works every day in the real world. People are exceptionally resilient. People move that inch when common sense tells them that it can't be done. People do the smallest thing they are able to do and then move it another step forward again. Hope shines through.

Because we are so used to going to the doctor, getting a prescription and getting better, we are surprised that the key to change is us. Maybe psychological approaches aren't really like medicine. They are more like physiotherapy. When we go to the physiotherapist, we are given the tools needed to improve. They can show us where our bodies are struggling, where and why we are feeling pain. Then we can begin to strengthen areas that are hurt and build our bodies back up in order to engage and enjoy the world around us. When we go to the psychologist, we are given the space and guidance needed to recover. But the work comes from us.

We can address our thoughts. We can begin to see these little bursts of neural electricity as they are. Not some universal truth but vague interpretations of the world around us. In the words of St Paul, '*We see the world as through a glass, darkly.*' Not some perfect truth but a snapshot of the world from a limited perspective. If our thoughts are critical and negative, we can step back and ask: why? Do they have to be like that? Are they even realistic? Are they an accurate interpretation of the world around us?

Our emotions are often the sea on which our body surfs. From one perspective they can seem dangerous and cruel; from another, they can take us to dizzying heights of enjoyment and pleasure. We have to know how to ride the wave. We have to know how this ocean beneath us works, and understand both the simplicity of its physical basis and the complexity of its psychological drives.

As conscious beings, we can step back from what we do. We are not automatons who can only act and react in a certain way; still, we often get stuck in damaging patterns of behaviour. Routines are difficult to step out of. We are not computers. We can change what we do. We can choose a different path even when that seems difficult to us. We can learn new ways of being that no one ever taught us and which we have never tried. The middle section of this book focuses on how to overcome unhappiness. We don't have to wait for a crisis. We can include these skills in our everyday lives, now.

HOW TO CREATE A HAPPIER COUNTRY

No man is an island,
Entire of itself,
Every man is a piece of the continent,
A part of the main.

John Donne

Often when we talk about mental health, we talk about what is inside the person. If they would just be different then they wouldn't feel the way they do. And that is true: what is inside the person matters. But there is also a larger context. We are not separate from our environment, our economy, our society.

The way the world is organised makes a difference to our mental health. From major factors such as being employed, to day-to-day factors such as access to childcare or the length of our commute, how our country is organised has an impact on our happiness. We live in a world that pushes us to be a certain way. If there is a global financial meltdown, as there was in 2007, then it's going to have an impact on our emotional well-being.

There are a couple of unlikely dreamers in the London School of Economics. They've asked the question: 'what if we didn't try to improve our economy and tried to improve the nation's happiness – Gross National Happiness – instead?' As a country and as a community, what would we prioritise then? What would you prioritise? Flexible working hours? Access to green space? Increased or decreased salary? What would matter to you?

This isn't in conflict with our economy. We need jobs. Poverty is one of the most reliable causes of unhappiness. So the economy needs to function well in order to offset this. But an economy is not a society, and a functioning economy is not the same as a functioning society. We, the community, create that by the choices we make and by the things that we prioritise.

When we look at the factors that underscore unhappiness in a population, poverty is the second biggest cause. So it's essential that we deal with poverty accordingly. But what is the number one predictor of unhappiness? Mental health difficulties. One in three people will have a mental health problem in their lives. Seven hundred and fifty thousand people have a mental health problem in Ireland today. The government estimates that mental health problems cost €11 billion per year. So if we want to improve the happiness of the nation, we need to improve the mental health of the nation.

There is an apocryphal story that the phrase 'to go round the bend' comes from the fact that all psychiatric hospitals were outside the town, hidden from the main road. The car carrying the patient literally went round the bend until you couldn't see it anymore. We in Ireland were very good at hiding the problem, but it didn't go away. In fact, it created long-term difficulties and a host of euphemisms: people 'suffered with their nerves', 'had a bit of temper' or 'enjoyed a drop'. The reality of people's suffering was hidden away with an untold cost on children, families and the community.

Everyone thought their family was the odd one out, so the secret had to be hidden. In fact, the truth is, at some time or another, every family suffered. Imagine a village that lived in silence even though every family was living through the same thing. Thankfully, attitudes are beginning to change. Yet stigma remains a major issue. Ireland is still that village.

I wonder if this post-crash generation will view mental health issues differently. Will they be viewed as normal health problems that aren't stigmatised, but as treatable and short-lived? Mental health has often been considered as something that happened to someone else, somewhere else. But we as a community are beginning to understand that this happens to people like us, people in our families. The way mental health is thought about and talked about in society makes a difference. Stigma is a small word with large real-world ramifications. It can mean people failing to seek support from colleagues, as workplaces are far from conducive environments in which to broach the subject. Moreover, mental health services are consistently the last to be funded.

It is a commonly held belief that medication and hospital admission are the only possible ways of treating mental health difficulties. These beliefs are at least a generation out of date. There are robust, reliable short-term psychological treatments that work; there are strong, community-based social interventions that work. Medication is imperfect but evidence-based and effective. These treatments could be available to all should society choose to prioritise them.

We need to promote prevention strategies; early intervention services; services focused on young people; easily accessible, low-intensity treatments; a psychological focus rather than a biological focus; and community-run services. All of these will save lives in our localities. All of these will treat mental health problems quickly and effectively. All of these will improve the level of happiness in our country. None of the fears of yesteryear need affect lives today.

There is a strong agenda informing us that our illnesses are ours alone to deal with. But if we don't start examining the system in which we live and ensure that suitable safety nets are in place for those who need them, when they need them, then we will never be able to shift from individual solutions. Those dreamers in London are professors of economics. They don't dream of a utopia. They see the grounded facts that if we wanted to seek out the goal of Gross National Happiness, we could do it. But that is a quiet, slow revolution that extends far beyond the psychology clinic. It involves every house and every family stating categorically that our happiness and our children's happiness matters. That would be quite a revolution.

CONCLUSION

The body you inhabit is sixty thousand years old. The reason it survives is down to its capacity to adapt. We adapt to challenges, grow and learn, and then grow and learn again. This process never ends. Our ability to change is intrinsic to our human nature. This is why we should never lose hope. We are built to change. I am in the privileged position of seeing that people can and do change, every day. Therapy is the process through which the seed of hope, which is in every person, is nurtured and allowed to grow. These powers of change, adaption and growth may not be easy to channel. However, by taking up the challenge we can begin to understand the nature of what it is to be human.

Change to the Power of Three

Biology gives you a brain. Life turns it into a mind.
JEFFREY EUGENIDES

What causes mental health problems? Everyone experiences stress at various points in their lives, but a much smaller proportion of us experiences significant mental health problems; there is a major difference between the two. There is often a lot of confusion surrounding subjects such as stress, anxiety, worry or depression. Each and every one of us will be sad at times in our lives, but only 10 per cent of us will have depression. Each and every one of us will be stressed, but only 8 per cent of us will have an anxiety disorder. When people working in mental health talk about issues such as depression, they mean the diagnosable condition as opposed to the unavoidable daily pressures or emotional setbacks that are part and parcel of life. However, one-third of us will have a significant mental health problem in our lifetime. Most of us would like to be able to deal with these problems before they become severe enough to warrant a diagnosis.

When people talk about experiencing mental health difficulties, they talk about their lives slowly diminishing: everything is harder; ordinary things are painful. Mental health difficulties like these are powerful; the distress is overwhelming and it significantly interferes with day-to-day life. Depression and anxiety are mental illnesses that can be costly and debilitating. In the old days, we didn't talk about mental health and we didn't record it officially. If a family member had pronounced mental health difficulties, they were often bundled away to an institution. Suicide wasn't recorded by the coroner. Psychological problems are now part of common parlance but do we actually know what is going on?

When we think about what causes mental health problems, most professionals speak about the 'bio-psycho-social' model – the biological, the psychological and the social. Professionals from different backgrounds will emphasise different parts of the model, but most accept that mental health difficulties are caused by an interaction of the three. Bio-psycho-social factors are often discussed separately as if they are different worlds. They are treated as if your brain isn't part of your body or your psychology is floating off somewhere else in the room. You'll notice this in the media. Headlines will shout, 'New gene found for depression' or 'Economic recession leads to suicide', but the key to understanding mental health is that these three factors interact. How our body works will have an impact on how we feel; how we feel will have an impact on our social worlds (work, relationships, etc.); our social worlds will affect our neurochemicals and so on. The cause isn't a straight line; it is circular.

In this book I focus on psychological treatments for mental health problems and so have very little to say in the area of medication. There have been controversies about how commonly antidepressants are prescribed, their side-effects, and whether they are as effective as claimed. These controversies are well explored in other books. My own personal experience is that medication can often be useful, especially when used alongside talking therapies or other approaches. It is impossible for therapy to work if the person is so depressed that they cannot get out of bed to come to sessions. If someone is so anxious that they struggle to interact, then it is hard for them to make the changes needed to improve. Most GPs I meet would love to have options other than prescribing antidepressants but they know there are six-month or year-long waiting lists for access to psychological treatments. There's no major problem with prescribing medication per se; the main issue is a lack of access to other forms of treatment.

People often look at mental health problems as a mountain to climb and wonder how they can overcome such a challenge. But because of the interplay between the biological, the psychological and the social, there is every reason to be hopeful. Each positive step you take in one area will have a positive impact on every other aspect of the circle. Improve your exercise regime and it will improve your mood. Tackle negative or anxious thoughts and it will have a positive impact upon your relationships. Make a positive change in your social world and it will improve your thinking. Change to the power of three.

BIOLOGICAL

People often ask the question about mental health: 'Is it all in my mind?' And the answer is 100 per cent yes and 100 per cent no.

We often separate our bodies from our minds, but of course the two are inextricably linked and so the biological is going to have a large impact on how we feel. Everything that is intrinsic to our body is going to have an impact on our emotional equilibrium. People often wonder whether or not there is a physical component to mental health. Although there is a lot that isn't known and much research yet to be done, there is no question that mental health problems are deeply biological.

Everything we experience is filtered through our brains. If you have a cramp in your foot, it is experienced by a nerve and processed in your brain. The meaning you bring to it comes from your mind. How worried you are about the cramp will depend on whether you are lying in bed or running in the Olympics.

GENETICS

Genetics matter. I am five foot ten and have blue eyes. This is because the men on my mother's side are five foot ten-ish and have blue-ish eyes. My face, my voice, my heart, the diseases of which I am at risk, are all going to be influenced by my genes. I'm relatively fit, have a healthy weight, run three times a week and yet have the cholesterol of a seventy-five-year-old man. This is due to my genetic make-up.

There is a significant body of research which shows that genes play a role in mental health. If I have family members who have had a mental health problem then I may be at increased risk. It is less clear if genes play a role in specific diagnoses but there is very little doubt now that our biological make-up is important.

There are a few aspects of this worth considering. Just as everyone has a family member who has had heart difficulties, everyone has a family member who has had mental health problems. This is because they are really common illnesses. Given the number of scientific discoveries about the importance of genes in the last decade or so, we can often be fooled into thinking that genes determine our 'health' at every level, both physically and psychologically. Of course, this is not true. Genes are part of the story – but only part.

For instance, identical twins have identical genes. If genes were the only factor in causing mental illness then it would follow that if one identical twin had depression, the other twin would be guaranteed to have it too. Yet this is not the case. If one identical twin has depression, the other has only a 37 per cent chance of having depression.

The risk is higher than average but it is significantly lower than it would be if genes caused depression. All the things that happen in your life are going to have a significant effect on whether you develop depression, as well as genes. No one is doomed to depression.

Since genes are the one thing we can't control, we can only look at all of those factors that we do control.

Often the discussion about the causes of mental health difficulties devolves into a heated 'nature vs nurture' debate. However, new studies are focusing on the interaction between nature and nurture on the understanding that neither one of them tells 'the whole story'. Research indicates that our life experiences and our genes interact in a complex way. What happens if we are at increased risk of depression and experience a trauma? What happens if the trauma occurs when we are very young and our brain is only developing? What happens if we take cannabis or other substances and already have a genetic predisposition towards depression? What happens if we experience small, repeated stresses over a long period of time? What happens if we didn't develop positive emotional attachments when we very young? Genes are important but they are not the whole story.

I have the same difficulties with cholesterol that my grandfather had but I have a better diet, better knowledge and better healthcare. What happens to me is going to be influenced by all of these things, and the outcome I have is likely to be utterly different.

NEUROCHEMICALS
Good moods are caused by four brain chemicals: endorphin, dopamine, oxytocin and serotonin. It would be nice if they just flowed all the time. But they were NOT designed to do that. Your happy chemicals were meant to do a job. They turn off when the job is done.
Loretta Graziano Breuning, *Meet Your Happy Chemicals*

Neurochemicals are organic molecules that participate in neural activity. They take all the messages from the outside world and create an internal world for us. They are the bicycle couriers of the brain. There are hundreds of such chemicals and we only have a good understanding of a few.

Endorphins developed to help us manage pain. When we exercise or escape from danger, endorphins kick in to help us manage the discomfort of the physical effort. But when we don't need them, endorphins don't flow.

Dopamine is released as a feeling of reward. Generally this happens before we actually receive a 'prize'; you might have noticed that sometimes the anticipation is better than the prize itself. In this way, dopamine motivates us to pursue long-term goals, even if they take a considerable amount of time to achieve.

Oxytocin is the basis of the feeling of trust. All animals release oxytocin when they're born. This allows them to develop attachments to their mother. In childhood, oxytocin is stimulated when a mother holds her baby. In adulthood, oxytocin is released when we have a sexual experience with someone.

Serotonin is probably the best known of all neurotransmitters because it is the basis of Prozac and a whole family of antidepressants. They are known as SSRIs (Seretonin Specific Reuptake Inhibitors). In everyday life, serotonin flows when we feel contented, confident or safe, as opposed to feeling hopeless or helpless.

A question people often ask is 'why don't we experience "happy" neurochemicals all the time?' Sadly, it would lead to disaster. If endorphins flowed all the time, we would not notice ordinary, but important, everyday aches and pains. If dopamine flowed all the time, *everything* would have significance and meaning. If oxytocin flowed all the time, you would trust people you shouldn't trust. If your serotonin levels were high all the time, you'd constantly feel over-confident and superior to those in your social circle which is hardly a recipe for healthy relationships or friendships.

These are the neurochemicals that psychiatric medication is centred on but they are also the neurochemicals that are triggered by exercise, sex, trusting relationships, positive outcomes, developing meaning and a whole host of positive occurences that we can bring into our lives. We don't want these neurochemicals to be artificially low. We need the motivation and pleasure that they bring, but we need to live a life that allows the natural ebb and flow of happy neurochemicals and that sets off these chemicals naturally.

SUBSTANCES

The substances we put in our body are very important. We know this inherently. If you are used to having a cup of coffee or a cigarette at a certain time, try putting it off for an hour. How do you feel? Cranky, more anxious, less able to cope, not quite yourself? Miss a meal or two and see what happens to your mood. Our mood and our ability to cope are very quickly affected by the inputs to our bodies. And these are just minor chemicals that we miss for a short period of time. How we feel is intrinsically connected to what we put in our bodies.

Alcohol is going to have an enormous impact on mood. Most advice around alcohol is concerned with addiction and physical health problems. As a result it's recommended that men drink no more than seventeen units a week and women fourteen. But even a much lower level of alcohol has a strong effect on our mood. Think about it. One or two glasses of wine can make you feel happy. That's why we drink it. But we also know people for whom one or two glasses of wine can make them feel sad. Again and again, we find that people with mental health problems are particularly susceptible to negative sensations as a result of ingesting only small amounts of alcohol. Chart it out. What was your lowest point this week and was it in the forty-eight hours after drinking? People can make their own choices around this but it is important to know what impact alcohol has on your mood. It can vary greatly from person to person. There is a large group of people who, though they don't exceed the recommended number of weekly units, find their low mood or anxiety are exacerbated by alcohol.

COGNITIVE FUNCTION

A key aspect of mental health difficulties that we sometimes neglect is brain function: attention, memory, emotion, decision-making. Our understanding of brain function has come on in leaps and bounds over the last twenty years. It is still not as precise as we would like, but we have a much stronger understanding of how it works. Attention, memory and concentration all play a significant role in depression and all have their underpinnings in brain functioning. People with mental health difficulties complain that they often struggle with these functions when they are unwell, but they return to normal when they feel fine.

People report:
- Overly negative or distorted thinking
- Difficulty concentrating
- Distractibility
- Forgetfulness
- Reduced reaction time
- Memory loss
- Indecisiveness

This reduction in efficiency of the neurological processes is one of the most common frustrations for people with mental health problems. To everyone who says that mental health is just in the mind, these can be deeply frustrating biological processes that people with mental health difficulties confront. They experience great difficulty in concentrating on work or in school and find that their memory is not as sharp. This makes their day-to-day functioning harder. It is easier to make mistakes, and the sense of 'not-being-oneself' increases.

We are beginning to learn how the nature of these functions has an important role to play in mental health problems, for instance depression. When we are depressed we have an attentional bias towards things that are negative. We focus squarely on the worst possible scenario and fail to take account of the greater picture. If ten people give us feedback, it is human nature to gravitate towards the worst piece of criticism. When people say that everything seems blacker when they are depressed, that is entirely true on a technical level. Their brain will be paying attention to all the negative facets of their environment, at the expense of all the positives. If everything you see and everything you remember is negative, then the whole world seems a much darker place. Exactly the same thing seems to happen with anxiety, but instead attention and memory are biased towards threat. Similar patterns can be observed in different diagnoses around fear of rejection, embarrassment or paranoia.

We don't understand the process in all of these cognitive changes. Which comes first, the depression or the cognitive bias? The interaction between how our brain functions and how we feel is going to be important when it comes to developing treatments over the next ten to twenty years.

PSYCHOLOGICAL

We are not just our brain – our mind is as important. This book is grounded in the Cognitive Behavioural Therapy (CBT) model of how the mind works.

There are many therapy options that people can explore. Some focus on relationships, some on experiences in childhood or our family structure. Over the last forty years, CBT has become the most widely used therapy of its kind in the world. CBT is based on the idea that our thoughts, feelings and behaviours feed into each other. When our thoughts become negative, they can create a vicious cycle of negative behaviour and low mood that's difficult to break out of. It's not rocket science but it is really important to understand because it tells us something that seems counterintuitive. The best way to feel happier is not to focus on our feelings, but to change what we think and what we do. Think about that again. The best way to feel happier is to focus on what we *think* and what we *do*. OK. Let's go feel happier.

Common sense suggests that there's a cause and effect dimension to our emotions; something happens and then we have a feeling about it. It's my birthday; I feel happy. I fail my driving test; I feel frustrated. CBT is based on the idea that we have a thought in-between the event and the feeling:

- I fail my driving test …
- I have the thought: '*nothing ever goes right for me*' …
- I feel frustrated …

These thoughts fly by so quickly they can be hard to even notice. But we can catch them and we can reflect on them and we can check them against reality. If we seize the negative thought, we can alter our perception:

- I fail my driving test …
- I have the thought: '*many people fail the first time, I'll get it next time round*' …
- I'm not over the moon but nor am I too upset …

The ability to catch and reflect on our thoughts is a key skill in maintaining our own happiness. You have thoughts whizzing by all the time. They might not be true. They may be partly true, half-true or sometimes true, but we often believe a thought as if it is an objective 'truth'.

Some of the most common thoughts those with mental health difficulties mull over include: 'I have no friends'; 'I'm not good enough'; 'I don't deserve to be happy'. Notice the pattern of these thoughts. They are often short: 'I am not …'; 'I should not …' They are rigid. There is no flexibility in them and they are quite generalised. They don't allow room for other perspectives or experiences. CBT asks us to see if we can create flexible thoughts that reflect the complexities of the world around us.

Our thoughts and our feelings are not an end in themselves. They lead to our behaviour.

▸ If I have the thought: *'I'm going to hate the work night out on Friday. It's a total waste of time …'*
▸ I'm going to go to the night out but I mightn't get involved …
▸ What's guaranteed to happen? I'm going to have a terrible time and I'm less likely to go next Friday …
▸ It will reinforce my original thought: *'It's a total waste of time'* …

In this way, it is a self-fulfilling prophecy. Our behaviour reinforces what we already believe, whether that belief is 'true' or not. This reinforcing behaviour happens in relationships, in work, in sleep, in our social lives. We do things that reinforce our negative beliefs and, by doing so, the reality of the situation is completely ignored. If I want to change how I feel, I'm going to have to change what I do and what I believe.

There are a small number of natural, negative emotions that are part and parcel of life: anger, sadness, grief, shame, anxiety. However these feelings can easily become overwhelming. When we have an experience that we find painful we often try to dismiss it and distract ourselves or pretend it didn't happen.

These are a few examples of ways people avoid dealing with emotions:

▸ Ignoring their feelings
▸ Overeating
▸ Excessive alcohol consumption
▸ Misuse of recreational or prescription drugs
▸ Avoidant behaviour, e.g. exercise, shopping, sex
▸ Constant intellectualising and analysing
▸ Overworking

Do you recognise any of the above? There's a good chance that if you do, then behind them are emotions that are difficult to process. What happens if we just stop the behaviour? We start to be upset by the emotion and that is, well, upsetting. But we also learn that emotion isn't permanent, it is transitory and we are much more capable of dealing with it than we believe. We only learn to manage the emotion when we allow ourselves to feel it.

An emotion will come and go because it is evolutionary in basis. Its purpose is to give us information ('this is painful, unpleasant, dangerous'), to increase sensitivity to our environment ('this place is safe, this place is unsafe'), to allow us to build relationships ('I love this person'; 'I am frightened of that person') and, most importantly, emotions are a short cut towards action. Anger pushes us towards violence and defence; sadness pushes us towards withdrawal and self-protection; anxiety pushes us towards escape.

These actions are all short term. They are designed as a brief burst of energy and over the course of an hour or so gradually come back down. When we block negative emotions, we don't get the information we need. We learn something that is untrue: 'I need to keep busy to cope', and the emotion never gets the opportunity to resolve itself. It is a kettle that keeps on boiling. The behaviour becomes the problem. It keeps dampening the emotion and then setting it off again. If we never get to feel our anger, it just bubbles under the surface and pops out at the worst possible time. If we never feel our anxiety, then it never gets the opportunity to be relieved.

Often by not engaging with the main emotion, we get caught up in lots of minor emotions. Instead of feeling angry, we feel ashamed. Instead of being anxious, we feel low or powerless or overwhelmed. Paradoxically, suppressing emotion doesn't decrease the amount of emotion we feel – it increases it. We end up with complex emotional reactions: angry about being anxious; guilty about feeling sad.

CBT examines those vicious cycles of thoughts, feelings and behaviours that people may experience. The psychologist and the client talk through different stressful or negative situations and try to identify some of the underlying features. Then we try to discover the most common negative or anxious thoughts. Do I believe 'I'm useless' or why do I think 'I can't cope'?

It's amazing how little we 'think' about our thoughts and what positive change can occur when we start to examine them. Once we've achieved this we can look at any behaviours that might be unhelpful or reinforce our negative thoughts. CBT asks the client to change; to test out new behaviours; to take small steps to see what it is like doing something else. Using these behavioural changes, the client builds new thoughts about the world and their place in it.

When you combine these steps in a compassionate way, remarkable things happen. People see themselves in a whole new light and begin behaving in entirely new ways.

SOCIAL

What happens in our world has an enormous effect on how we feel. The biggest predictors of depression are social occurrences: divorce, unemployment, financial strain, bullying, isolation. Our social world and our environment have a huge impact on how we feel and whether we are going to become anxious or depressed.

It is also the area that brings us the most happiness. Love, marriage, friendship, trust, attachment. These are the factors that people say are the most fulfilling in their lives. Yet relationship difficulties are the number one predictor of depression. This is very understandable. The people we are closest to are the people we spend the most time with; the people who have the biggest impact on us; the people whom we want to love and to be loved by. If a stranger doesn't understand us, it doesn't make much of a difference but if our partner doesn't understand us, it hurts. The stress brought about by relationship difficulties can be particularly persistent and challenging. It brings about uncertainty. It challenges who we think we are. It challenges our sense of being loveable. It challenges our past, our present and our future. Of course it is going to have a dramatic effect on our outlook.

We have just experienced one of the most severe economic meltdowns in modern history, with an attendant increase in the rates of anxiety, depression and suicide. Generally one bad event doesn't make us psychologically unwell. It is the unrelenting repetition of negative events – be they related to unemployment or financial pressures – that does the damage. Activities that would normally operate as stress relief, such as holidays and nights out, gradually become curtailed. Freedom and choice get eroded. Every month, it becomes a little bit harder and optimism becomes a little more dulled.

There are two key risk periods for the development of mental health problems: from ages fifteen to twenty-five and from ages sixty-five to seventy. These are two periods of major transition. Young people find themselves moving out of the structure of family and school, while facing the challenges of having to live independently, maintain and develop romantic relationships, and use alcohol in a mature fashion. The stress of fitting in and, for some, not fitting in have a huge impact on our sense of well-being. This is obvious in the prevalence of news reports concerning the link between cyberbullying and suicide. Every day, throughout schools up and down the country, children will become anxious or low if those peer relationships are challenged or if they find themselves isolated.

For older people, the transition from the working world to the third stage of life marked by retirement poses huge challenges. Houses that used to bustle with children become quiet. People who have been preoccupied for much of their adult lives with the demands of the nine to five often find it difficult to fill their days once retirement becomes a reality. As such, they have to find a new sense of meaning and a new routine. This often occurs at the same time as age-related illnesses or physical setbacks become an issue.

INTERACTION

The key to understanding mental health difficulties is the interaction between biological, psychological and social. How our body works will have an effect on how we feel; how we feel will have an impact on our relationships; our relationships will affect our neurochemicals and so on.

For instance, it is very common to lose sleep because of worry. This has a biological effect in that it disrupts our circadian rhythms. It has a psychological effect in that we then spend most of the night worrying about not sleeping. When we go into work in the morning, it makes concentrating more difficult and is more likely to lead to a difficult day. When we go to bed the following night, we are more likely to worry about why we can't sleep. Each area interacts with the others and it is easy for a vicious cycle to be formed. The opposite is also true. If you do something worthwhile or rewarding and something starts working for you, then it has a positive impact on everything else. For instance, if you can get your sleep right, suddenly you have more energy, you have less time to worry and you feel more confident that you can address the challenges each new day presents.

We can talk about it and we can think about it but the key step will be doing it. Take one aspect of this 'bio-psycho-social' model that looks useful and bring it into your life. Because these aspects interact, taking one step has the potential to impact upon every other aspect of your life. One positive social step will help us both biologically and psychologically. Change to the power of three.

How to Be Happy

An Apple a Day

One cannot think well, love well, sleep well,
if one has not dined well.
VIRGINIA WOOLF

It is strange to think, but sometimes we have to teach ourselves how to be happy. It doesn't come to us naturally. Children know how to do it, but priorities and expectations often take over for adults. There are thousands of different advice columns telling people what they should do to be happy. My personal opinion is that it doesn't really matter what the advice is. Pick one thing and just do it.

For that to actually happen, you will need: a diary, a pen, post-its, a calendar, a wall chart, a fridge magnet, a reminder beep on your phone and every app that ever existed. This is because as human beings, we are not very good at changing our habits. We get stuck in ruts and it can take us decades to get out of them. We are creatures of habit – often bad habits. We say we are going to go on a diet. Nothing happens. We say that we will start going to gym. We go half a dozen times and never go again. Half the country has the same hobby: losing weight. It is very difficult to change a habit but this is what we have to do. We have to look at what habits make us happy.

Most of us have got into the habit of ignoring our mental well-being. We think that everything else is more important. I want to get back to walking but I can't this week because of blah, blah, blah and I can't next week because of yada, yada,

yada. Everything is more important that our well-being. Well, this simply isn't true. We have to prioritise our own well-being because *nothing* happens if we are not well. Most people's gut response to this is: 'I want to but I couldn't possibly.' I couldn't do it because of family or children or work commitments. My response is always this: 'you have to.' Everything else depends on your well-being: your family, your work, your children. If you are not well, then everything else falls apart. Your responsibilities require you to be well. So your health has to be the priority and that, of course, includes your mental, as well as your physical health. The amazing thing about all of this is that when we do prioritise our health, everyone copes. They all find a way to manage. We think that if we took five minutes off the world would collapse around us but this simply isn't the case.

There is a great organisation in the UK called Mindapples (you can check out their website at mindapples.org). They have a very simple message. We know that we need five portions of fruit and veg a day to stay healthy. Well, what are the five things we are going to do for our mind on a daily basis? Any five things. There is no point in eating all the fruit and veg on one day and ignoring it for the rest of the week. What are you going to do for your mind every day? You already know some of the things that would be helpful, but I would bet pounds to pennies that you are putting them off.

What are the sort of things we are talking about? TCS: Total Common Sense. More exercise; proper eating; going to bed earlier; reducing how much we try to squeeze into a day; meeting friends and *really* talking when we see them; tackling some of the things we have been putting off; tackling some of those goals we want to achieve; taking fifteen minutes out and being quiet, just quiet.

So if I am going to start breaking the habits of a lifetime, how to do it? Try this:

1. Pick a realistic goal.
2. Now make it slightly smaller.
3. Put the time and place where this is going to happen into your diary.
4. Go through the diary for the next six weeks and make sure that you will be able to do it every week.
5. Record each time you do it in a diary.
6. Record how you feel when you've done it.
7. No matter what you do, compliment the effort. You did a quarter of the walk you wanted. Excellent. You only did it on half the days you initially hoped for. No problem. That's perfect.
8. Keep it up.

Turn the page for an outline of how the diary might look. The best way to use this diary is to try to build a balance into your week. There will be work, so where is the relaxation? There will be time alone, so where is the social time? Everything we do needs to be done with a sense of balance.

	MORNING	AFTERNOON	EVENING
MON			
TUE			
WED			
THU			
FRI			
SAT			
SUN			

One of my heroes is the economist Richard Layard (you can check out his website actionforhappiness.org) who has spearheaded a social movement to try to increase the level of happiness in society, primarily through encouraging people to take positive steps to improve their own sense of well-being. His researchers came up with ten different approaches to improving happiness based on really sound research involving large samples of the British population. The list is far from comprehensive but is still a pretty good place to start.

For the most part these are common sense pointers that we are all aware of; things your granny could have told you. But contrast your granny's advice with the demands of the modern world: working harder, being more isolated, the pressures of being young, the loneliness of being old, the pace of constant connectivity. We know what would make us happy but there is a reasonable chance that we are not doing it. We know what common sense tells us but there is also the sense that the world is moving in the opposite direction. Although society may promote pleasure, it is probably moving us away from happiness. We have to work quite hard to include some of the following in our lives – but that is key. The more we work on some or all of the following, the happier we'll feel.

Layard's ten suggestions are:

1. Relating to other people
2. Giving
3. Exercising
4. Appreciating the world around us
5. Trying out new things
6. Being goal-directed
7. Finding ways to overcome negative experiences
8. Increasing positive emotions
9. Acceptance of ourselves and the things that happen to us
10. Finding meaning

I am going to discuss in this and subsequent chapters how to go about incorporating these suggestions into your day-to-day life. You don't need to do them all and you don't need to do them all the time, but increasing how much time you devote to these pursuits will increase your opportunities for happiness.

RELATING TO OTHER PEOPLE

Many philosophers, neuroscientists and evolutionary scientists believe that people are intrinsically social creatures. In the words of Martin Buber: 'I am intrinsically you-ward.' Our orientation is towards other people.

Humans didn't survive sixty thousand years of evolution alone. We hunt in packs. We live in tribes. We raise children in communities. All of these collective efforts protected us from danger and, because of this, social contact has become hardwired into our systems. The brain has a very interesting way of working. When we do things that are good for us – exercise, good food, sex – it makes us feel good. As most people will agree when we do things socially, we feel good about it.

When we play on a team or work together to achieve a goal, we generally feel good. Think of Italia '90. Think about the atmosphere in the country at the time and the sense of connectivity to our neighbours epitomised by the shared colour of our jerseys. We can't always recreate the excitement of Italia '90 in our lives, but we can try to make sure that we are meeting and talking to people every day, in small ways and in large.

Loneliness and isolation are major problems in Ireland. It is most noticeable among the older generations but how many teenagers feel isolated? How many people move from office computer screen to TV screen, without a single meaningful human interaction to punctuate their day? From our earliest infancy, we are programmed to seek out faces and to look for the emotion in them. Throughout our lives, we are influenced by the emotions of the people around us. There is very good evidence that when we interact with a happy face, we ourselves become happier. Happiness is 'contagious'.

In the business world, people talk about 'face time' but in fact this is an important concept for all of us. When we are starved of interaction, it has a major impact on our mood. Imagine doing your current job without any contact with colleagues, customers or other people. That's eight hours with no interaction, the reward being a cheque at the end of the month. There is a fair chance that we would hate that job, even though the 'work' aspect might be exactly the same as we currently do.

My fondest memories of school aren't of the classroom, but of the various team sports that I took part in over the years. My fondest memories of college are of the societies I joined and, of my twenties, the relationships I formed. This isn't accidental; this is how we are hardwired. When we compare societies in different time periods and cultures, we notice that nearly every one has a hermit or a priest caste who live at a remove from the community, but they are the exception not the rule. Their importance in societies highlights how much the rest of society is connected. I don't know if Hillary Clinton is a great philosopher but when she quoted the African proverb, '*It takes a village to raise a child*', she hit on a fundamental truth of how humans are structured. We do better when we are together.

Yet increasingly we work in offices and cubicles. We drive alone in cars. We are absorbed by the screens on our smartphones during our commute. Without any effort, it is quite easy to spend large parts of the day in a bubble. Even when we sit together, how connected are we? Do we talk over the dinner table? Do we watch TV together? It is easy to be lonely in a crowded room. We have to make an effort to form a real connection, to have a real conversation. We have to make an effort so this one encounter has some real meaning. The busyness of our lives and the noisiness of our world means that our connections are really very precious and need to be both nourished and defended.

GIVING

Being social and giving are intrinsically entwined. One of the ways that we develop connections with others is giving, be it time, money or attention. Making the choice to give something of ourselves. Many neuroscientists and evolutionary scientists believe that people aren't just social, they are prosocial. We don't make connections just by pointing ourselves at people. We make connections by sharing ourselves with people.

You will recognise the sensation of walking past a homeless person and feeling guilty for not putting something in the cup. The body's response is immediate. We sense it in our gut: negative feelings kick in. The same is true for positive actions. If we visit a relative we haven't seen in a long time, we often feel good about it, regardless of whether or not the actual event was enjoyable. The way we build relationships is by small acts of kindness. We bring our partner flowers. We buy our friend a scarf. We chat with our neighbours. We remember birthdays and Christmases. Giving is how we build bonds, and bonds make us happier.

We cement relationships within groups by sharing experiences, be they positive or negative. How many teams and groups are built by being together in a time of adversity? Kindness given in a time of need is seldom forgotten. We are safer, happier and more likely to survive the trials and tribulations of life when we are in a group, and our genes and neurotransmitters know this. As a result we often feel a sense of reward from giving.

Yet it is easy in the modern world to feel cynical, to feel cut off. Sometimes other people's suffering is so overwhelming that we have to pull away. There is something very human about having to turn away from the suffering we see around us. We walk past a homeless person because we can't give to everyone.

We can't feel everything but sometimes that leads to our being cut off from *everything*. That cynicism leads to isolation and impacts upon our own happiness. We have to decide what we are going to allow ourselves to feel. What charity is my charity? What action in the world will be my action? I don't have to do everything but I do have to do *something*.

Like the discovery of fire, the internet has the potential for great harm and great good. One of the most positive aspects of it is the development of random acts of kindness. People, not restricted by border or nationality, can do something worthwhile for a complete stranger. The internet has been a vital tool in this regard. Last year, the Ice Bucket Challenge swept through the world. For those who don't know, this is a challenge to pour a bucket of ice water over yourself and donate towards a local ALS (Amyotrophic Lateral Sclerosis, often referred to as Lou Gehrig's Disease) charity. Before the Ice Bucket Challenge idea took off, ALS was a little-known disorder. Afterwards, it gained worldwide recognition and millions of euro have now been raised. This phenomenon is really important psychologically because it shows that we don't have to know the person to get a positive benefit from giving. In fact, we don't even have to have a pleasant experience (being doused in ice water is no one's idea of fun), but we still get a positive feeling. There is a sense of happiness that comes from giving, even to people we never meet, suffering from a disorder we don't understand. It is built into our fundamental sense of self and we feel happier when we do it.

APPRECIATING THE WORLD AROUND US

Many sensations give us pleasure. In fact sensation might be the quickest way to pleasure. The smell of fresh coffee; the taste of good food; the sound of brilliant music. All of it can fill us with joy.

A couple of months ago, I was on a meditation retreat in a beautiful part of Wales. I remember floating in a lake between two mountain peaks. I recall being so surprised by the strength of the emotion it evoked. I was doing nothing, but I was doing nothing in a beautiful place and I was open to seeing it. The sheer experience of living can bring great happiness, *but* we have to give ourselves room to enjoy it. I would never have had that experience in a normal working week, even in the same place. I had slowed down enough to experience it. The busier we are, the harder it is to notice the things around us. If we rush from the bus to the office, we never see the beauty of the architecture. If we hurry from task to task we never see the scenery. 'Stop and smell the roses' is an old cliché but that doesn't make it untrue. I live in Dublin, a city surrounded by mountains. A couple of weeks ago, I realised I hadn't been hillwalking in months. I had got caught in head-down-don't-look-up mode.

It is extraordinary what we prioritise in any given day. Generally it is the micro rather than the macro. We focus on the smaller events rather than on the larger processes. Recently, an audience gathered to watch *Dead Poets Society* to remember and commemorate the life of Robin Williams. At a key moment of the movie, the audience spontaneously stood and shouted, 'Oh captain, my captain'. For many there, it was an overwhelmingly emotional moment. They experienced what the Portuguese call *saudade*, a suffering you enjoy. This isn't an uncommon event. We only start to appreciate something or someone when they are gone. How much more important is it to experience something while it is still there? But for that to happen, we have to prioritise appreciation over efficiency. We have to give ourselves the space to experience all the emotion that appreciation brings.

Exercise
See 'Get the Body Right' (p. 65) for some helpful advice on the importance of exercise.

TRYING OUT NEW THINGS

We often spend our lives tied up in routine. There isn't much pleasure involved, nor is there much pain. It is anaesthetising. But there is a reason that humans didn't cease evolving in the caves and didn't cease with the bow and arrow, nor cease with fire. We are naturally curious. Christopher Columbus didn't know whether he would fall off the edge of the Earth or not, but he went to find out. Saint Brendan, a thousand years before, made the same journey to find out. We will risk hardship, danger and disappointment just to find something new. Discovering something new is part of who we are and it is important to our happiness.

There is a great satirical website called The Philosophers' Mail. It looks at tabloid stories through the eyes of professional philosophers. A recent story on *The X Factor* had a picture of Simon Cowell, and was captioned 'Ennui, on a jet ski'. Infinitely rich, on a jet ski, and infinitely bored. While it is an obvious dig at the super wealthy, it could also be a dig at any of us living lives of relative privilege and who are desensitised by routine. I remember as a child being taken on a day trip to Dublin Zoo. At that stage the polar bears were in a small enclosure with only a small pool to swim in and their food provided for them at regular intervals. Even to a small child they looked depressed. Animals that were used to roaming, to hunting, to challenges and novelty were emotionally bereft. The zookeepers there have very different strategies now designed to stimulate the animals. To this end they now hide the food from the monkeys within their enclosure. This means that the monkeys have to work to find it. It is always in different places. Rewards that we really work towards have a much greater impact than those we readily receive without effort.

Do we fall into the same trap? Often our jobs are repetitive: at a desk or in an office. Often our roles are repetitive: putting the kids to bed, filling the dishwasher. Spaghetti on a Tuesday. Curry on a Wednesday. It is very easy to fall into the trap of doing the same thing every day. These tasks may be quite pleasant in many respects but if nothing changes then we stagnate. We don't vary what we do. We don't seek to take something on. Change seems too challenging. We'd prefer to stay in. Stick with the routine. There is a balance to strike here but ultimately, as human beings, we crave variation and novelty.

Try this. Everyone washes every day. Do it differently. Reverse what you do. Choose to take a bath instead of a shower or vice versa. Pick a really pungent shower gel or shampoo. That's about as basic as change gets but notice how different it makes you feel. If you drive to work, try walking instead. If you already walk, try choosing a different route. Listen to a different radio station in the car. Buy different foods in the supermarket. Get out the recipe book. What does Jamie Oliver suggest you eat today? Give it a go. Now think of something bigger. This evening. This weekend. This isn't about spending money. It is about spending time, on ourselves. Galleries, museums, libraries, parks, beaches, mountains, forests, talks, lectures, friends' kitchen tables – all are free and easy to access.

Experience something new every day. It won't come to you. You have to go out and find it. It is about being Christopher Columbus in our own world.

BEING GOAL-DIRECTED

We've talked a lot about the 'here and now', but one of the things that gets us through difficult routines is the knowledge that it will pay off. We need to know the route will take us where we want to go. We study for the Leaving Cert in order to go to college, not because we love study. We jolt around the car park because we want to get our driving licence, not because we love car parks.

If we don't have medium-term and long-term goals, it can be a tough slog through dull or difficult tasks. We can keep ourselves motivated for work if we think that there might be a promotion, or if we know it will pay for a holiday. It is much harder to do it if we feel we are not progressing along a defined career path, or if our work goes unappreciated.

Sometimes we are so focused on the long-term plan that we neglect the short-term, day-by-day goals that keep our motivation buoyed up. Humans are funny animals. We do very well with the carrot but very badly with the stick. If our only motivation is that we *have* to do something then it is very easy for it to slip away.

So sit back, have a think about what your long-term goals are. Give yourself a bit of time, space and a pen or pencil. What would you like to have achieved in five years? What would you like to have achieved in one? Start sketching out some ideas. Nothing is set in stone. Just begin to think about what you would actually like.

Now what are your short-term goals? What would you like to achieve this week? How does this tally with the long-term picture? Does it move you in the right direction?

What are the short-term rewards for the small achievements? We need the carrot now. What is your incentive this week?

I am training for a ten kilometre run at the moment. That's the long-term goal. Fitter, happier, healthier, all of that. But it means I need to run a minimum of three times a week. So what is the small reward every time I run? This took me a while but it turns out, it is the route. I can run ten kilometres in any direction, five kilometres away from my house and five kilometres back; however, only one route takes me to the sea and affords a stunning view of Dublin Bay. This is the reward. I make small variations to the route every time but I always get to see Dublin Bay when I reach the halfway mark.

We often have aspirations but we seldom translate them into goals. Wanting to be rich won't make us rich, for instance. We need something more specific. Aiming to increase your income by 10 per cent over the next twelve months allows you to start planning and problem solving your way to achieving that. If you'd like to spend one night away in a guesthouse in Ireland every six weeks, start working out how you can achieve it. Want to be happier? Less stressed? Well, what are you going to do to make it happen?

It is amazing how once your goals become specific, they become so achievable. Things that people have talked about for years suddenly start happening. Lots of your life happened because you set a goal and got there. Exams, jobs, relationships. There's evidence of this all around us. Want one more piece of evidence. The book you are holding in your hand started out as a specific goal.

Finding ways to overcome negative experiences
See Chapters 6,7,8 and 9 to see how to deal with negative feelings such as depression, anxiety, worry and emotional dysregulation.

Increasing positive emotions
This is the chapter!

ACCEPTANCE OF OURSELVES AND THE THINGS THAT HAPPEN TO US

Whatever life may be, it certainly isn't smooth. One of the most important ways of maintaining happiness is to understand how to manage difficulties and unhappiness. What do I do when I lose my job? What happens when I am under stress? What do I do when I lose a loved one? I am going to deal with this throughout the book, but one of the key factors is acceptance of life's setbacks.

A strange thing happened in the world over the last fifty years. People began to believe that they should be happy all the time. Positive philosophies have a lot going for them but there is also a downside. Implicit is the belief that if you were stronger, better, worked harder, then you could be healthy and happy all the time. But sometimes reality won't be positive and that's simply a fact of life.

If we expect to be healthy and happy all the time, what happens when we are not? The core of this expectation is unrealistic. Sometimes we are not healthy and it is not our fault. Sometimes we are not happy and it is not our fault. We have seen a huge rise in levels of unhappiness because of the recession. The ground shifted under our feet and circumstances became much more difficult for everyone. Blaming ourselves or feeling guilty isn't going to help.

In modern western culture we are concerned with looking to the future and striving for more, at the expense of the here and now. The antidote to this is acceptance and transience. The acceptance that I am experiencing the things that I am experiencing and that in time they will change. 'This too shall pass' is a perfect adage for understanding the world. This wise phrase – quoted by King Solomon, medieval Persian poets and Abraham Lincoln – is built on an acceptance of who we are and where we are. We can recognise that we want something to be different. If we lose our job, then we recognise that we didn't want this to happen but there is also an importance in accepting that it happened without fault or blame or anger. It happened. This is the situation I am in. I'm not happy in this situation. I am grieving for something I have lost, and am furious because something has been taken. But it will pass. It may be positive or it may be negative but it won't stay the same. This is the nature of the world.

This isn't passivity. It is an active engagement in what we have because it mightn't last. We seek out pleasure in the people and things we have now. Equally, it recognises that suffering, though it may exist in the present, won't be the same in the future. It is an understanding, as imperfect as any day may be, that we are living it now and we should seek out what any moment might bring.

FINDING MEANING

When I consider my grandparents, I see how their lives were immersed in meaning. Religion was unquestioned; politics were clear; patriotism was universal. Family. Work. Parish. All of these institutions were venerated. They relied on them and they received a lot from them. There has been an extraordinary change for subsequent generations. Those touchstones of meaning have shifted. Now we each have to seek our own personal meaning in a world that is increasingly complex. Yet the things that we need, the things that we want, aren't that different from those of our grandparents. Most people would like to be in a permanent relationship; most people would like to have children; most people want a secure job and to be part of a caring community. We ask the same as our grandparents, but we have to find our own individual answers. That can lead to a lot of confusion and stress for people.

When Freud wrote about what makes us happy, he emphasised the need for two things: *lieben und arbeiten* (love and work). We need people to love us – whom we can love in return – and a role that gives us a sense of satisfaction. These are core components for happiness and when we lose one or both through a break-up, redundancy or our children leaving home, we have to strive to find a new way of fulfilling them.

Research also tells us that although love and work are important, if we have a sense of being part of something larger, this increases our sense of happiness even further. Is there a cause that we can commit to? A community that we can embrace and that will embrace us in turn? In our busy lives, it can be hard to set aside the time for such pursuits, but it is worth it. In Ireland, we are still strong on community spirit. If you drive past a football pitch on a Saturday morning, you still see dads coaching the under-nines. Bake sales, charity collections and school concerts are still well attended. These events build ties within a community and highlight our sense of ourselves as not being alone in the universe but part of the whole. That leads us to feel safer, warmer and less isolated, especially when we go through tough times.

Can we go 'larger' than just community? Can we find meaning above work, family or community? Victor Frankl is a famous Jewish psychologist who was imprisoned in Auschwitz. In his key work, *Man's Search for Meaning*, he detailed how vital larger meaning is in our ability to transcend difficulties and find solace in even the most appalling circumstances. He looked at all the people around him in the concentration camp and saw who survived and who didn't. He believed that fundamental to our ability to survive, even in the worst possible situation, was having something to live for and to truly believe in.

He saw meaning as personal and unique. We each need an individual framework through which we can view the hardships and joys of life. We need to find it, develop it, in our true selves and really know it. This asks major questions of us. What do we believe in? What is important to us? If we had to leave behind our normal lives, what would we take with us? Within the confines of our own heart, if we had to abandon everything, what would we hold on to?

This sense of meaning is vital to our happiness and vital to our ability to come through unhappiness. Having survived three years in Nazi concentration camps, Frankl came to his philosophical conclusion that even the most absurd, painful and dehumanising situation has the potential for meaning. We don't have to overcome suffering to find meaning, we can find it anywhere at anytime. In fact some of the greatest meaning in our lives comes from the darkest moments:

> We stumbled on in the darkness, over big stones and
> through large puddles, along the one road leading
> from the camp. The accompanying guards kept
> shouting at us and driving us with the butts of their

rifles. Anyone with very sore feet supported himself on his neighbour's arm. Hardly a word was spoken; the icy wind did not encourage talk. Hiding his mouth behind his upturned collar, the man marching next to me whispered suddenly: 'If our wives could see us now! I do hope they are better off in their camps and don't know what is happening to us.'

That brought thoughts of my own wife to mind. And as we stumbled on for miles, slipping on icy spots, supporting each other time and again, dragging one another up and onward, nothing was said, but we both knew: each of us was thinking of his wife. Occasionally I looked at the sky, where the stars were fading and the pink light of the morning was beginning to spread behind a dark bank of clouds. But my mind clung to my wife's image, imagining it with an uncanny acuteness. I heard her answering me, saw her smile, her frank and encouraging look. Real or not, her look was then more luminous than the sun which was beginning to rise.

A thought transfixed me: for the first time in my life I saw the truth as it is set into song by so many poets, proclaimed as the final wisdom by so many thinkers. The truth – that love is the ultimate and the highest goal to which Man can aspire. Then I grasped the meaning of the greatest secret that human poetry and human thought and belief have to impart: the salvation of Man is through love and in love. I understood how a man who has nothing left in this world still may know bliss, be it only for a brief moment, in the contemplation of his beloved. In a position of utter desolation, when Man cannot express himself in positive action, when his only achievement may consist in enduring his sufferings in the right

way – an honourable way – in such a position Man
can, through loving contemplation of the image he
carries of his beloved, achieve fulfilment. For the
first time in my life I was able to understand the
meaning of the words, 'The angels are lost in perpetual
contemplation of an infinite glory'.

Victor Frankl

Frankl's wife, Tilly, was murdered by the Nazis in Bergen-Belsen concentration camp in 1944.

Understanding our own suffering brings meaning to the darkest corners of our lives. Having a framework to understand the vicissitudes of life allows life to be meaningful. Our sense of meaning will change throughout our lives. We can find it and refind it again, infinitely. The important thing is to seek. The world has changed a lot since 1943. Our busy world hides its meaning under brands and commodification. Yet true meaning exists just below the surface. So it is all the more important to drive ourselves towards a greater commitment to finding meaning. Our happiness depends on it. The human race has searched for meaning as long as it has existed. There is great wisdom in every philosophy and in every religion if we are willing to search for it. We need not be concerned with the complexity and sophistication of modernity but with very simple things. Finding, holding, embracing and committing to something bigger than ourselves. When we look outside ourselves, we become stronger. Happiness is not an abstract concept. We build it in both large and small actions. It is easy to ignore or neglect until we turn around and find we have lost it. It is something to be cherished, sought and guarded. But firstly we must decide to seek it out. We must decide we want to be happy.

Get the Body Right

To get back my youth I would do anything
in the world, except take exercise, get up early,
or be respectable.
OSCAR WILDE

The image of the perfect human body is thrust upon us everywhere: the ideal youth sells us hoodies; the ideal mom sells us cleaning products; the ideal man sells us tools. Magazines. TV. Billboards. We cannot get through a day without looking at someone else's perfectly toned physique.

Yet we often don't think of our mind as being part of our body, in the way we do our heart, our lungs or our liver. One of the keys to happiness is understanding that we are human machines. We can do extraordinary things: paint the Sistine Chapel, climb Mount Everest, sing an aria. Yet, it is vital to our happiness to understand that we are also machines: that we need to refuel, that we physically break down. We cannot do everything we think we should do simply because we believe we should do it!

Treat the human body right and we feel better. Treat it badly and we feel worse. I have a very good friend who told me this story. She was walking home from work one evening and rang her fiancé several times; when, after numerous attempts he still hadn't answered, she left a really irate voicemail wondering why he was never there when she needed him and explaining that there was something important that she needed him to do and to call her back immediately. Then something dawned on her: she had salad for lunch that day. Something else dawned on her: the last time she had had a fight with her fiancé she also had salad for lunch. What was going on? She wasn't eating enough carbs. She was working really hard. She was trying to do something positive by eating a light meal but there wasn't actually sufficient carbohydrates in her lunch to sustain her until six o'clock. This wasn't about her. It wasn't about her fiancé. It was about an unbalanced diet.

The relationship between our bodies and our emotions is really interesting. For many people, certain emotions can be a warning light that something is wrong with their bodies. They become tearful, grumpy or stressed when their body is tired, hungry or overtaxed. The answer to that is not psychology. It is pure biology: put the body right. Often our emotions are the best indicator that something is out of sync with our lifestyle, routine or diet. The easiest place to effect change is in the body because it will respond directly to good food, exercise and care. My friend didn't need years of therapy to work out her relationship issues. She needed a carb-based treat! We often rush to psychology and miss basic biology. Get the body right.

WHERE ARE OUR BODIES AT?

It is really important to remember that our bodies are expertly crafted, multifunctional machines, but they were not designed for the modern world. Our design is based on our experiences as a species, and most of that experience has been deeply physical: hunting, gathering, farming. The office environment of the late twentieth and early twenty-first century presents new challenges and, in terms of human evolution, our bodies aren't designed for it.

We are the most stationary generation in history. Think of your grandparents: they walked, they cycled, they worked on farms or in factories. Think of our lives: we sit in a car, we sit in an office, we sit in a car, we sit at a dinner table, we sit on a couch, we go to bed. Even if we throw in the occasional trip to the gym, it hardly redresses the imbalance. Our backs weren't built to sit for eight hours at a time. Our eyes weren't built for screens. Our brains weren't built to engage with two phones, two email accounts and a Word document all at the same time. Our bodies are resilient and can manage these pressures, but only up to a point. And when our body doesn't like something it responds with negative emotion: pain or stress or a lack of energy. Our mood can definitely affect our body, but our body also affects our mood. It is a circular relationship. One of the most obvious ways of offsetting the damage is to do something good for our body.

EXERCISE

We are human machines built for activity. Our brain rewards daily activity and punishes inactivity. Maybe it is surprising but exercise has some of the most positive outcomes of any intervention for depression and anxiety. Too much inactivity has a negative effect on our mood, and a moderate amount of activity has a very positive effect on our mood. When we think of the chemicals involved, it is not hard to see why. Exercise reduces the level of adrenalin that is a key chemical in anxiety. It increases the production of endorphins that improve our mood. It makes us physically tired, thus improving our sleep, and it can give us a sense of achievement which is good for our self-esteem. So exercise simultaneously increases the production of happiness hormones as it reduces the production of stress hormones. As a result we can feel more positive about ourselves.

We need a minimum of thirty to forty minutes of exercise per day. This should match our level of fitness, while pushing us a little. For some people, it will be a brisk walk. For someone else, it will be a five kilometre run. When we push ourselves a little bit, the brain calls for back-up and we get a boost of endorphins. This dulls any pain and gives us a mild 'high'. It is only when we push our body a little beyond its comfort zone that we get this specific chemical response.

Endorphins are a key chemical in our experience of happiness. They are naturally occurring, non-addictive and have no downside. Why wouldn't we want them? In fact, they are the sort of chemical that we need more of, and exercise is the most straightforward way of attaining them.

There is, of course, a balance to be struck. It is becoming increasingly clear that too much exercise is bad for us but, frankly, there are few of us in the western world for whom this is a problem. Like all interventions, we are looking for the happy medium. A little and often beats extremes of too much or not enough.

There are many psychological benefits to exercise, and chief among them is increased self-confidence as a result of feeling fitter and healthier. We can set goals and have a sense of achievement as we tick them off. Exercise can be a deeply social activity which allows us to enjoy the company of others. Five-a-side football, running clubs, walking clubs, yoga classes and gyms allow us to develop our social circles. At a basic level, these are simply fun.

Yet we have to admit that we often don't want to exercise. We know we should do it; we just don't really want to as it can be difficult to find the motivation. It is an effort at the beginning of most sessions and this is the point at which most people tend to give up. They cut it short or just avoid it all together. I was chatting to someone recently who told me she paid €50 a month in her gym. I couldn't believe it could be so expensive. She said it isn't; it's actually one of the cheaper gyms in Dublin – it's just that she has only gone twice in six months. The process of some pain for some gain underscores our relationship with exercise. But it will reward you when you put the effort in and it will reward you every time.

The fact that we often don't want to exercise is exactly why good routines and habits are vital. These are the things that will carry us through on the night we just don't want to leave the house. If I always run on Tuesdays, then I'm more likely to go this Tuesday. If I have a class booked on Thursday then I'm more likely to go on Thursday. That is even more true if someone else is counting on me. If we can link up with other people, we are more likely to do it; the company is likely to carry us through the first few difficult minutes when we want to cop out, and it makes it a lot more fun.

Many people say they are exercising but they don't see the benefit. Generally this is because they are putting in the effort but not quite enough, or not quite often enough, to get the reward. This is a real pity because they are putting in lots of work without getting the 'goodies'. A little additional effort brings a lot more benefit.

Many people ask how, as a psychologist, I contend with the distressing emotions, traumas and difficult stories I come across every day. There's a two word answer: fifteen kilometers. I run five kilometers three times a week. On the weeks when work is light, I do less. On the weeks when work is heavy, I do more. It is absolutely key to staying on an even keel. Like everyone else, I have slips when the weather is particularly bad or I'm feeling lazy, but it has an immediate effect on my stress levels. My job stays the same but without the run, I feel more anxious.

DIET

Before we do anything complex, we need to make sure the basics are in place. Are we eating too much? Are we eating too little? Are we eating frequently enough? You would be amazed at how many people don't eat enough or don't eat at the right times. They do all their eating in the evening but all their living/working during the day. The old saying 'eating like a king at breakfast, a prince at lunch and a pauper at dinner' has a lot of truth to it. But generally when you look at people's diets, it is the reverse: barely anything in the morning, a rushed lunch and then overeating at dinner. And you don't feel great? Well, no surprise.

What happens when we start to get stressed or are very busy? We skip meals. We add more caffeine and sugar to our diet. This won't work because our bodies are machines that need careful maintenance. Developing a poor diet often arises as a failure to prioritise our own well-being and putting any other priority ahead of it, as if self-sacrifice makes us more efficient rather than less. The first sign that it isn't working? Our mood, often a more nuanced marker of undereating than hunger, deteriorates.

When we are under pressure, we solve our dietary problem in all the wrong ways and generally opt for the quick fix. This is fine now and again but it is a disaster if it becomes a long-term arrangement. We add three 'uppers' to our diet: caffeine, alcohol and sugar. All of these give us a boost. They are world's cheapest drugs. Everyone feels better when they take them but almost everyone has the same reaction to them. What comes up, must come down. So the greater the lift, the greater the drop. One cup of coffee? Fine. Two? Three? Four? What's going to happen to our bodies when they are bombarded with stimulants? They don't make us more efficient; in fact, we end up channelling our inner Hunter S. Thompson.

We get a short-term boost and a long-term crash. The more frequently we do it, the less efficient we become. Some of us remember as students pulling all-nighters in which we mainlined sugary energy drinks and coffee. We managed this for a week or so leading up to exams but, as adults, many of endeavour to do this all year round by working long hours and depending on the same stimulants to keep us upright. It will work for a while until your mood becomes compromised. You will become stressed, cranky, emotional and less efficient.

We need to eat whether we feel like it or not, and we need to eat more (and better) when we are busy. It doesn't matter whether you have to do it, feel like you should do it, have a deadline or anything else. You need to eat or everything else stops working.

IDENTIFIED DOWNTIME

We have to embrace the idea of being a machine at our core. What would happen if you ran your car twenty-four hours a day? It wouldn't last long. You'd burn out the motor. Look at the speedometer in your car. It might go as high as 200kph. But we don't drive the car at that speed, just because we are able to. Why? Because we know exactly what will happen. We'll crash it or it will burn out. Exactly the same thing happens to us. It doesn't matter if it is paid employment or work in the home or a combination of the two. We can keep pushing ourselves. We can work harder and harder, for longer and longer but it always ends the same way: crash or burn out.

Like any machine, we need rest. There has to be adequate time, every day and every week, for us to recuperate, refuel and recharge the batteries. We know when we work. It is laid out for us in our contract. Our week is organised around it. But when do we stop? This is often a much more haphazard affair. We probably get two weeks in summer and a week at Christmas. But other than that, our rest time is often left up to fate. If something comes up, we often sacrifice our downtime. We get less rest for reasons such as:

‣ A busy period in work
‣ Issues with childcare and family
‣ Housing or DIY crisis or car crisis
‣ Friends or family crisis
‣ Key times of the year.

In fact, there is probably no week in which something doesn't come up that eats into our allotted downtime. That is because we don't really prioritise rest. We seem to think of ourselves as infinite resources that can never be tired; this simply isn't true.

What we are is extraordinary. We have an extraordinary ability to create. We also have an extraordinary ability to recuperate, but we don't use it as well as we should. We need to prioritise it, to guard it carefully and to only give it up in the most serious of crises. We need to organise our week around it. Make sure that money, time, babysitters are all utilised to achieve it. We need to be ruthless about recuperation and not squander it.

It doesn't matter what we use to recuperate. We have talked about exercise, but equally it might be watching an episode of our favourite TV show or enjoying the company of friends. It might be a movie or weekly date night. It might be a long bath, a good dinner, a lovely walk, a quiet coffee, a loud nightclub. We don't need to be to 'clean' about it. Fun matters too. Breaking out of the routines matters. As the saying goes: 'All things in moderation, including moderation.'

My work diary is laid out meticulously. At the moment, I can see my appointments running two and three months in advance. But I am lackadaisical about organising my downtime. We only need to bring the same professionalism that we bring to our work calendar to our recharge time. Book it in advance. Don't double book. Don't leave it to fate. When downtime is respected, everything else flows.

HIGH PERFORMANCE ATHLETES

When preparing this chapter, I tried to think about who does these things best. I thought about the old boss of mine who booked one night away every six weeks, and booked the next break the instant he came back. I thought about all the friends I know who are committed to their tag rugby and five-a-side soccer. But the people who personify this best are professional athletes.

If we can adopt some of the organisation athletes bring to their lives, we can gain a lot. There are two key principles:

1. They understand that their bodies are machines; if the machine breaks down everything else stops. It doesn't matter how smart, how knowledgeable, how committed or how willing they are, if the machine won't do the job, the job won't get done.

2. Understand the law of diminishing returns: the more effort we put in, the more productive we become for a while, but after that, as we get more tired, the productivity diminishes. The best thing we can do when our output starts to dip is recuperate. That might be five minutes. That might be a day off. But adding recuperation make us more productive and more efficient, not less.

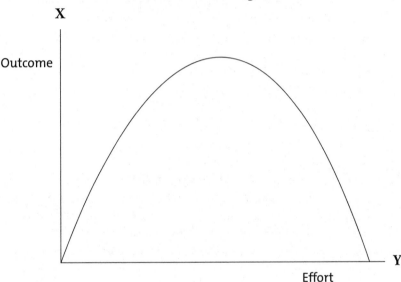

The Law of Diminishing Returns

X

Outcome

Y

Effort

Professional athletes think about their bodies in an entirely different way to the rest of us.

‣ They predict the pressures that will be placed on them. They will look at their year and see when the busiest times will be. For an athlete, that will be the end of the season but for an ordinary person, it might be Christmas. It might be the end of the financial year. It might be the sale season or the last week before holidays. Teachers know when their most difficult times are. So do doctors, nurses, police and firefighters. Businesses know their seasonal changes. Athletes also predict the toughest times of their week. For them, it is the match day or the track meet, and they organise the week around it. Again, most of us can examine the week ahead and know which days are the busiest. It usually isn't hard to predict when stress is going to arise.

‣ Athletes do something we don't. They prepare. They organise their sleep, their diet, their exercise and their recuperation in order to manage this busy period as well as they can. We often stoically grit our teeth and try to get by buoyed up on coffee, clinging to our mental health by our fingernails. With a small amount of organisation we would get through these periods much more easily. What's more, the athlete is able to do this on an ongoing basis, whereas our performance gradually gets ground down.

‣ Athletes peak. They work as hard as they can in order to achieve the goal and then they stop. Work isn't infinite. It is goal-driven and then has an end point. I recently heard that part of the regime in the Munster rugby team involves coaches monitoring players to ensure they don't overtrain halfway through the training week, because it is the wrong time to peak. Players are tapped on the shoulder and told to step out in order to conserve their energy. Yet how often do we work through lunch, skip breaks, work into the evening or do task after task at home without a breather? This doesn't make us more efficient, it just tires us out.

‣ Athletes put huge effort into recuperation. They spend the day after the match taking ice baths or receiving physio or studying videos to enhance their performance. They sleep and rest. They don't train for a couple of days. They recognise that recuperation isn't weakness but the most efficient way of achieving what they want to achieve. Brian Cody, the most successful hurling manager of all time, once spoke following an All-Ireland final which ended in a draw. He had two weeks to prepare before the replay. Was he going to have his guys out running sprints the following Monday morning? No, he replied. He was planning to prescribe a week off before resuming training.

Rest is a vital component of efficiency. I've never met anyone who doesn't have time to take a little more rest. I've met people who believe they don't have the time. I've met people who are addicted to the busyness and the constant bustle, but I have never met anyone who can't find some extra time to rest. And guess what? They become more productive as a result.

SLEEP

One of the primary symptoms of stress is a disrupted sleep pattern. People can end up oversleeping or undersleeping. We all know how difficult life can be if our sleep is disrupted even a little.

Every person's sleep cycle is different and every person's domestic situation is different. In this section, I try to give some general advice on managing sleeplessness. There are a number of key lifestyle factors. As much as possible, it is important to have the same bedtime each night. No two people's routines and demands are the same. Shift workers will be different to nine to fivers. Breastfeeding mums will be different from college students. Generally the evidence suggests that we keep the same routine most nights of the week. So if we go to bed at 11 p.m. and get up 7 a.m. we should try to maintain that routine throughout the week. It doesn't matter whether we sleep badly the night before or not. Always try to get up at the same time. If you get up at 7 a.m., always get up at 7 a.m., whether you have had a good sleep or not. If you start pushing back your wake-up time then gradually your bedtime will also start to shift. Don't sleep in the afternoon, no matter how bad your night was. It will only make it harder to sleep the following evening.

There is no nice way to say this: our bladders are really small. Sometimes we need to pee. The amount of liquid we take in during the evening has to go somewhere. The older we are, the more of an issue this becomes. So we have to be okay with getting up in the night. We also have to manage how much liquid we consume in the evening. Sometimes you meet people and the last thing they do at night is have a hot drink, be it tea or cocoa, but it has to go somewhere.

We need exercise in order to fall asleep. We might be emotionally tired, we might be mentally tired, but unless we are physically tired, we won't sleep. The first thing we examine in the clinic when someone isn't sleeping well is their exercise routine.

We all know about caffeine. Caffeine raises your heart rate and has an impact hours after you've consumed it. Most Irish people only think of coffee when they think about caffeine. They don't think of tea. Generally the rule is that coffee has a rapid effect but tea often has a slow-burn impact, still affecting people hours afterwards. As a general rule, Irish people drink coffee by the cup but they drink tea by the pot.

Alcohol is relevant in lots of different areas in this book because of its powerful biological and psychological effects. How do we know that it is powerful? Well, we all know people whose personality can change after two glasses of wine: the person who becomes aggressive; the person who becomes incredibly tearful. We know it impacts upon our driving and our accuracy. Most people also recognise that it impacts upon their sleep. Everyone's body has a different relationship with alcohol, but lots of people will recognise the quick-to-doze, quick-to-wake pattern. They are asleep on the couch by eleven o'clock but tossing and turning all night. Like everything we've looked at in lifestyle factors, it is about looking at our own patterns and figuring out what works and what doesn't work for us.

We often find that TV helps us sleep. Generally, it seems that screens (iPads, laptops) and smartphones do the opposite. The quality of the screens, plus the proximity with which we hold them to our eyes appear to have a stimulating effect. A very interesting modern phenomena is that of would-be sleepers being kept awake by mobile phones placed near their beds. That sense of anticipation at the prospect of receiving incoming texts or updates keeps us half-awake and slightly on edge.

It is generally thought that there is good and bad bedtime behaviour – and this refers to adults just as much as children. No two people are the same, so each person will have a different routine. Generally, we need the last hour before going to bed to be a period of repose. We need to be gradually slowing down, not taking on anything too emotional, taxing or stressful. The routine should stay pretty much the same: put the cat out, put the dishwasher on, lock the back door, wash our teeth. We are getting our bodies and our minds ready to sleep. Bedrooms need to be fairly tidy. Beds need to be comfortable and the temperature needs to be right. Pillows and mattresses need to be of a good quality. We can get into bad habits of watching screens in bed, but generally the best thing to do is to reserve bed for sex and sleeping.

THE PROCESS OF SLEEPING

You have to close your eyes. This may seem beyond obvious but it is amazing how many people don't do it, especially if they start getting frustrated that they can't sleep. (If you fall into this camp, try some of the tips below.)

When we are trying to sleep we want to concentrate a little, but not too much. If we allow our brain to wander, then it is likely to bounce into some topic that is interesting or worrying. Trying to think of nothing just doesn't work. We end up thinking about trying to think about nothing. What I have been recommending to clients recently – and there has been very positive feedback – is to try to watch a movie playing behind your eyelids. Let it be a movie that you know inside out, but preferably not a horror! Now very slowly, in real time, go through every scene. If it's *The Godfather*, say, picture the wedding: Luca Brasi learning his lines; Michael talking to Kate; Enzo the baker going into the office to see Vito. Gently concentrate on every detail. Keep going. If your mind wanders, gently bring it back to the next scene. This also works for TV shows or books, or any fictional scenario that is easy to picture and to remember.

WHAT TO DO IF WE CAN'T SLEEP

Many sleep specialists encourage patients who haven't fallen asleep within forty-five minutes or so to get out of bed. Go watch a little mindless TV or read a magazine. This isn't a battle. It's a chance to do something lazy and fun that you wouldn't normally do. Make sure you move to another room. You are aiming for twenty to thirty minutes of gentle activity. The key to this is your emotional reaction. Don't get annoyed at yourself or feel guilty about watching a little late-night telly; when the time has elapsed gently bring yourself back through your routine. Wash your teeth again. Go to the loo again. Fluff the pillows again. Fix the bed and gently go through the process of watching the movie behind your eyes again.

When I was a young researcher, I worked for one of the wisest psychiatrists I have ever come across. He and his wife had just had a baby and he was often up during the night as a result. From my own perspective, in my mid-twenties, being woken repeatedly every night seemed like a nightmare. However, I would see him the next morning at 8 a.m. for team meetings looking remarkably rested. When I asked him his secret, he told me: 'what could be nicer than standing in the moonlight, holding your son in your arms?' The perspective we take on sleep makes a huge difference to how well we sleep.

Worrying about not sleeping is the most destructive thing we can do. The more we worry, the more adrenalin courses through our body. The higher the adrenalin, the more difficult it is to sleep. The most common sleep difficulty people present with is worrying about not sleeping. Often as people go to bed, they will have thoughts running through their mind like 'If I don't sleep, it means I won't be able to cope tomorrow'; 'Not sleeping makes me ill'; 'Not being able to sleep is a nightmare'. By feeding in to this tendency for catastrophic thinking, we decrease the likelihood of sleeping well.

Then if we don't sleep we often get really frustrated. We toss and turn and get angry. We think of all the things that will go wrong if we can't sleep. We watch the clock with mounting annoyance: 3 a.m. ... 3:15 a.m. ... 3:25 a.m. Frustration is the enemy. Sleep is important but in order to achieve it, we have to trick our brain a little bit. Steve Davis was once asked how anyone could take part in a snooker world championship final without becoming anxious. His reply offers beautiful psychological insight: 'You have to do something as if you don't care, even if it is the most important thing in the world to you.' This is the same for sleep. We have to go to bed, not caring whether we sleep or not.

Here are some useful things to tell ourselves:

- 'It would be nice to sleep tonight but to be honest there are loads of nights I don't sleep. So it doesn't really matter.'
- 'I'll just do the second best thing. Rest, relax, be quiet.'
- 'Even if I don't sleep, I'll manage.'
- 'Tomorrow won't be perfect but it will be fine.'
- 'If Margaret Thatcher could run a country on four hours' sleep, I can manage on less than that.'
- If you are feeling very brave, recite the following mantra very slowly: 'I can't sleep and I don't care.'

We can see the whole system of how our body interacts to help us sleep. Our diet, exercise, downtime, everything has its role. We have to come to sleeping lightly. We can't bully ourselves to sleep. We can't worry ourselves to sleep. We have to gently bring ourselves to sleep as if we don't care whether it happens or not.

Mindful Living

The present moment is filled with joy and happiness.
If you are attentive, you will see it.

THÍCH NHÂT HẠNH

Mindfulness is a simple form of meditation that has been translated from Buddhist practice into the West over the last thirty years. It has been used to improve the lives of people with chronic pain, suicidal thoughts, depression and other significant difficulties. It asks people to pay attention, moment by moment, without judging.

When we think of mindfulness, we often picture monks in robes but it is an ordinary, grounded experience that anyone can try. A client of mine recently called it 'wakefulness' and I really like that. Because that is what it is: being awake to the world around you. We are often so consumed by our worries or distracted by daydreams that we are not fully connected to what is going on around us. How often does the daily commute go by in a blur? How often have we eaten something and barely tasted it? Mindfulness is about being awake to those moments. It sounds airy-fairy but it really isn't. Sometimes, we think of meditation as involving some alternative state of mind. Mindfulness doesn't ask this. It is about zoning in rather than zoning out.

In this chapter we are going to talk a little about mindful practice, but mostly we are going to talk about mindful living. There are lots of good books that will guide you through mindful practice. Mark Williams' *Mindfulness: Finding Peace in a Frantic*

World; Jon Kabat-Zinn's *Full Catastrophe Living*; Thích Nhât Hạnh's *The Miracle of Mindfulness*; and Tony Bates' *Coming Through Depression: A Mindful Approach* are all excellent books. But something I have noticed is that people often get so lost in reading about mindfulness that they don't actually do it. This is like reading about running. The best way you can learn to run is with a pair of trainers on. The best way of learning mindfulness is by doing it in a class.

The goal of this chapter isn't to teach you mindfulness meditation. Lots of other people can do that better than me. The goal of this chapter is to bring a little bit of mindfulness into everyday life. I also know that reading about mindfulness won't make us mindful. So I have structured this chapter a little differently. After every couple of paragraphs, there is a little mindfulness exercise designed to get us to stop and experience our current moment and prevent us from becoming merely passive readers. Each exercise should only take about a minute. As you read through, stop and do the exercise. Notice what you experience. You'll get a lot more from this chapter by taking the time out to do the exercises. In fact, you would get more from only doing the exercises than reading the chapter – but hopefully you'll do both!

There are two components to mindfulness: formal mindfulness practice and informal mindfulness practice. A formal mindfulness practice asks us to try to pay attention to something, and when our mind wanders to simply bring it back to that thing. We aren't trying to relax, zone out or stop thoughts. We are trying to zone in. It is a practice, and the point of it is to allow ourselves a few minutes in the day when we are free of distractions, just paying attention. There are a number of eight-week guided mindfulness courses available in clinics and centres around Ireland and this is probably the best place to learn. Mindfulness is best experienced, not thought about, so someone who will guide you through will be really helpful. After that it is about continuing those practices in your daily life.

Maintaining regular practice is tough. Personally, I go through phases: three or four really good weeks; three or four weeks where I do nothing. I've stopped giving out to myself about it. I know I'll come back to it. I enjoy it too much not to.

At this stage the meditation I like the most involves sitting in silence while paying attention to my breath. I have an app on my phone that sounds a mindfulness bell every five minutes during a meditation, encouraging me to bring my attention back to my experience. The garden has been really good for this over the summer but I haven't settled into an autumn routine yet. I'm lucky to have my own office in work. I regularly get ten free minutes towards the end of my lunch hour which I use for mindful breathing.

Informal mindfulness asks us to bring the skills of mindfulness to everyday life. So when we are writing a document at work, we concentrate on that task exclusively, without also checking emails or texts, jotting down memos or succumbing to other distractions. When we are with our kids, we are just with our kids. When we are eating an orange, we are just eating an orange. I've often been pulled up by my loved one over dinner because although I have sat down to eat, my mind is still in the office. If I was being more mindful, I would just be there. Just chatting, just talking, just listening.

Exercise

Close your eyes for a minute and listen to your breathing. [Really do it. I can see you are not doing it. Come on. How was that? Did you notice anything?]

Both formal and informal components are vital to being mindful. Notice that I don't say doing mindfulness. This isn't something to do and then get back to buzzing around like a bluebottle. It is about *being* as best we can, each and every day. It is about mindful living. Being awake to the world around us.

Exercise

Close your eyes. Rub your thumb against your middle finger for about thirty seconds. Pay attention to the sensation.

I find digital contraptions addictive. I simply can't resist opening a new email, even if I know it's rubbish. The ping of the little unopened icon is irresistible. Being mindful is about focusing on one thing at a time and appreciating it. It is deeply practical. Aspects of the Buddhist tradition have been integrated into many human pursuits from art to sport; in fact there are very few human endeavours where it can't bring improved focus. Now how do we bring mindfulness to emails and technology? Well, it is an open question. Here are some options: turn off the little pop-up icon; only use one piece of technology at a time; delete apps you know are distracting; when you have to get something done, leave all the other devices in another room.

Thích Nhất Hạnh is a Vietnamese Buddhist monk who has done a lot to bring mindfulness to the West. He is the head monk in a mindfulness community in France, called Plum Village, and wrote the influential book, *The Miracle of Mindfulness*, which I mentioned earlier. He is also a great calligrapher. A friend recently returned from Plum Village with one of his calligraphies. It says, 'Drink your tea'. That's it. Everything you need to know about mindfulness is in that short sentence. When you are drinking your tea, just drink your tea.

This is such a simple command that we might get annoyed by its apparent naiveté. We want it to be more complex. We want rules and steps and catechism. Mindfulness is about learning to pare back to the point that when we drink our tea, all we think about is drinking this tea, appreciating this tea, being with this cup in this moment. Then after finishing the tea, go and do something else.

Exercise

Go drink some tea. Slowly, quietly. Don't do anything else, just drink the tea.

Mindful living isn't passive. It isn't doing nothing. It is in fact very active. Rather than getting lost in our thoughts or doing ten things at once, it asks us to focus on one thing really well. After Buddhist monks, the people who do this best are snipers and professional athletes (especially those that take penalties or free kicks). We are not going to spend much time thinking about snipers, but imagine eighty thousand people in a stadium with their eyes fixed upon you. Imagine you have to take the penalty kick that will win (or lose) a match. What would be going through your head? Amazingly, those men and women are able to concentrate on just kicking the ball. Not on the crowds, not on the noise, not what it means to win and lose. In fact, what differentiates the very best professionals from their peers is not simply their skill, but their capacity for extraordinary concentration at the most difficult of times – including a World Cup final that would make the rest of us shudder.

Exercise

For the next minute, close your eyes and just listen to the sounds in the room.

There is a wonderful paradox to this. The more we pare back, the more we can engage with the thing in front of us. When we ignore the voices in our head, we are more effective, more productive and we enjoy things more. Simple things start to produce extraordinary pleasures. When we overload our plate with food, we end up feeling nauseous. When we focus on just one bite, it produces real joy.

Exercise

Go have a bite of a food that you like. Take a minute to eat and enjoy that morsel.

These exercises sound wonderful, right? What people don't tell you is that in the beginning, this is a right pain in the neck. You might feel relaxed but you might also feel anxious, twitchy, bored or self-critical. As you sit there, focusing on your breathing, there is a fair chance that your mind will be on anything *but* your breathing. It will be on work, home, the shopping, the kids. What happens in reality is that we get annoyed with ourselves: '*I'm meant to be focusing on my breathing and all I'm thinking of is that stupid meeting this morning. I'm the worst person ever at this. Maybe this isn't for me. Maybe I should just do something else. Zumba is meant to be good ... no zumba is stupid, why am I thinking about zumba, I'm meant to be thinking about mindfulness. Maybe pilates ...*'

It seems strange. We are trying to be quiet and relaxed, and yet our minds have never seemed so loud. Mindfulness doesn't ask you to explore these thoughts. We don't need to understand them. We don't need to think more. Only notice those thoughts and move back to our breathing.

In meditation we discover our inherent restlessness.
Sometimes we get up and leave. Sometimes we sit there

but our bodies wiggle and squirm and our minds go far away. This can be so uncomfortable that we feel it's impossible to stay. Yet this feeling can teach us not just about ourselves but what it is to be human … we really don't want to stay with the nakedness of our present experience. It goes against the grain to stay present. These are the times when only gentleness and a sense of humour can give us the strength to settle down … so whenever we wander off, we gently encourage ourselves to 'stay' and settle down. Are we experiencing restlessness? Stay! Are fear and loathing out of control? Stay! Aching knees and throbbing back? Stay! What's for lunch? Stay! I can't stand this another minute! Stay!

Pema Chödrön, *The Places that Scare You: A Guide to Fearlessness in Difficult Times*

Someone else experienced all of these thoughts too: the Buddha. When he wrote about meditating, he discussed all of the thoughts that got in the way of being able to meditate:

1. Desire: wanting it to be different: better, shorter, easier.
2. Ill-will: getting annoyed at yourself.
3. Tiredness: getting tired and zoning out.
4. Restlessness.
5. Doubt: becoming unsure that you are meditating correctly. Becoming unsure you are even meant to be meditating.

It is likely that you experienced some of these thoughts as you experimented with the exercises in this chapter. If you haven't experienced these thoughts, it is probably because you skipped the exercises. If you are thinking like this, then even in your very first meditation, you will be meditating just like the Buddha. If you experience meditation as a pain in the neck, you are not getting in wrong. You are experiencing exactly what everyone has always experienced.

Exercise

Stop for a minute and begin to notice the thoughts that are arising for you at this time.

If mindfulness is so annoying, why do it?

The Buddha famously said, 'life is suffering'. This wasn't because he was pessimistic or depressed. He recognised that there are difficulties everywhere. Suffering is a very loaded word in the West. What if we translated it as 'life is full of frustration'. Most people would be able to agree with that. If someone offered them a better way of working with life's frustrations and disappointments, they would be interested in that. For the Buddha, in order to be happy, there is something important about accepting frustration, not running away from it. Not fighting it because as soon as we fight frustration we become ... more frustrated. So this isn't about philosophy, it is about what works, what will lead us to being able to manage our day-to-day frustrations better. Much of the behaviour that undermines our happiness are ways of trying to avoid frustration. None of them work.

Mindfulness suggests something else: be with frustration and it will pass itself. It sounds paradoxical. It sounds like it couldn't be true. Nothing I say will be able to convince you. This is something you have to experience yourself. One of the purposes of formal mindfulness is to put us in a place of minor frustration so that we can practise sitting with frustration, and learning how quickly it passes.

Exercise

Take a short walk. Frame with your eye a few things you see, as if you had a camera. 'If I had a

camera, I would take a picture of that branch with
the light reflecting through it.'

You will experience the same five frustrations as the Buddha, and
you don't have to do anything about it. If you just continue to
meditate, they shift all by themselves. The point of mindfulness
isn't to avoid frustration but to accept it, be with it and allow it
to pass. If we sit with it, it will pass. Not just in the place where
we meditate but in every corner of our lives. In the beginning,
mindfulness is difficult, and that's ok; it's meant to be. But it
quickly becomes easier and more pleasant and from it we can
learn to manage frustration throughout our lives.

Exercise

Set an alarm for three minutes' time. Sit for three
minutes in silence. Maybe notice how frustrating
this is initially. Come back and do it again later,
seeing you how feel then. Come back and do it
again a little time after the again (three, three-
minute periods is not very much to ask). See how
it feels the third time.

Thinking like this can seem really strange to people. Surely we
should be trying to be positive? If we want to be happy, why
would we bring frustration into our life?

A strange thing happened in the world over the last fifty
years. People began to believe that we should be happy all the
time. Suffering was something we could defeat through willpower. If we tried hard enough, we could be happy all the time.
Never in the sixty thousand years that the human race has been
on the Earth have people thought that before. No matter what

continent we lived on, no matter what period of history we were in, people always believed that frustration was part and parcel of living. We have always believed in happiness too, but alongside negative feelings. Both came together: ying and yang, the black wolf and the white wolf, happiness and sadness. Then a generation or so ago this shifted. We came to believe that if we were just stronger, better or worked harder then we could be healthy and happy all the time.

What do positive emotions do for us? Well, the point is, they do nothing. Their very existence is a calming agent. Sunshine, lollipops and rainbows reduce cardiovascular activity. They drive behaviours such as curiosity and openness. We do silly things, we do pointless things and we do things with other people. A lot of the best things in life are silly, pointless and shared with other people. When we look at the physical health of happier people, their thinking appears to be more flexible and creative and their behaviours appear to be more varied. Researchers have found that positive thinking has health benefits including increased life span, lower rates of depression, greater resistance to the common cold and reduced risk of death from heart attacks.

Exercise

Close your eyes, slowly breathe in an out for a minute. Picture the ebb and flow of the sea with each breath.

This all seems very clear: happiness good, stress bad. Except it ignores reality. There *will* be stresses in life. We live in the world. We live with other people. We even love some of them. We will feel angry, sad and frightened. We were built to feel these things. They keep us safe and keep us from making the same mistakes over and over again. Negative emotions are hardwired. They are not an aberration from the norm. They are part of what it is to be human. In order to live with these emotions, we have to have a mindset that incorporates them into our lives somehow. Not 'I am never going to get stressed' but 'how am I going to be when I get stressed?'

Acceptance of the ups and downs in our lives allows us to manage life's frustrations. Often people believe that experiencing negative emotions is a sign of weakness or a personal failing rather than an entirely normal human experience. Seeing negative emotions as essentially useful allows us to tolerate them and learn from them. If we expect to be healthy and happy all the time, we often end up blaming ourselves or the people around us when we are not. We become frustrated at our own unhappiness. This leads to self-criticism and anger.

Exercise

> Notice what feelings you are experiencing right now. Breathe with them. Take three breaths.

Mindfulness suggests that there will be lots of difficulties in life; that expecting otherwise is unrealistic; that believing you will not be affected by them is unrealistic. You can't fight being angry by being angrier. You can't fight being frustrated by getting more frustrated. It doesn't work.

Being able to understand, accept, tolerate and bring compassion to the natural and normal negative emotions in our lives is a really important part of happy living. We can see our emotions and thoughts as the natural ebb and flow of the tide of human experience. They come, they go. We know one thing about our emotions for sure: they don't last. Can you remember how you felt an hour ago? Try to remember a thought you had two weeks ago.

We don't want to wallow in negativity, but noticing our negative feelings is a part of mindful living. If we ignore or suppress our negative emotions, they are much more damaging than the negative emotions themselves. The more we suppress them, the more they return. Grief, sadness and distress are part of our make-up. They are part of human existence. The way we live has to embody this. In order to be happy, we have to accept that sometimes we will be sad. Sometimes we will feel stress, but this is not a permanent state. Like all things in life, it is transient.

Modern western culture is based on striving for more and seeking more. With that striving comes worry. Should I do something different? Should I be different? The antidote to this is acceptance: an acceptance of who we are and where we are. We can work and change and grow and adapt but part of us also has to balance this with the scale of the world and our minuteness in it.

Picture yourself as a hiker at the base of a huge mountain. If we try to move the mountain, we will grow tired, frustrated and ultimately fail. If we accept the mountain as it is, we can conquer it. We may tire in our journey and need to rest. So rest. We may get frustrated at the climb. So feel frustrated. We don't have to pretend the mountain doesn't exist or that it is our fault for growing frustrated. We can accept the toughness of the climb and the difficulty we feel. With each step, the mountain will pass beneath us until it is no longer there and we are on flat ground again.

Exercise

Think of something that you don't like about yourself. Focus on it for a minute. Then gently say to yourself a few times: maybe this is just the way I am.

As we accept ourselves and the world around us, we can bring warmth to this. We are not looking to achieve some robotic state, never feeling, always distant and separate. When we think of mindfulness picture the Laughing Buddha, not Mister Spock.

We can bring a compassion to ourselves and to the people around us. Compassion asks us to be gentle and to hold things lightly. I remember discussing this with a mindfulness teacher of mine. I talked about wanting something very strongly: for the people I work with to get well. This seemed genuine and positive but it also often led me to be stressed and worried. She suggested holding this lightly. Not wanting something with an aggression but with a compassion towards myself and the people who come for therapy. Wanting doesn't have to be a battle. We can hold the things we want lightly. I've never forgotten the advice and try to bring it to work most days. I credit it as one of the reasons I haven't burnt out or become cynical about my work.

Exercise

Picture holding something you want. Picture holding it lightly, like a butterfly, in your hands.

This compassionate, warm and gentle approach is an important part of mindful living. Generally, we are very good at bringing compassion to other people. We can be kind and loving to them, suggest support and bring understanding, but when we suggest the same thing for ourselves, we are resistant.

Often mindfulness touches on a whole host of underlying beliefs about ourselves or the world around us. We have beliefs that we couldn't or shouldn't stop; that we can't relax or that we have to earn the right to relax; that we don't deserve compassion. People bring up a range of reasons why they shouldn't be compassionate towards themselves. They think something catastrophic will happen if they give themselves a break. It is a couple of generations since people thought 'spare the rod and spoil the child'. Yet that is often exactly the belief people bring to themselves: 'If I stop, I'll get soft or lazy; or I'll stop working altogether.'

Exercise

Take a quiet minute and slowly repeat to yourself: 'may I be happy, may I be healthy, may I live with ease'. Allow yourself a few minutes just to feel those words as you repeat them.

The strange thing about the exercise above is that it generally creates two contrasting reactions. On the one hand, people might enjoy it and find it warm and relaxing. On the other, people react really negatively to it. They find themselves becoming aggressive and reject it. This second reaction is really important to think about.

Why do we deserve love and compassion? Let's really ask. The question is not rhetorical. Why do you deserve love and compassion? Often people will say that they don't. They aren't a good enough person or there is something wrong with them, or that they have to earn it.

I think there is an answer. Why do you deserve love and compassion? Because you are a human being. An ordinary human being. You don't have to achieve it. You are a human being and every human being deserves kindness and empathy. Every religion recognises it. Every law defends it. Your intrinsic dignity is held just by being. You are deserving of love and compassion.

We can resist it. We can fight it. Maybe people in our past have made us think that it isn't true. Maybe we have told ourselves for years that it isn't true. That we do not deserve things that other people deserve. By your intrinsic humanity, you are as deserving of love and compassion as any other creature on the planet. Embodied in you is the fundamental truth of human dignity. But we can't ask that this love and compassion always come from someone else. No one is with us all the time, even our closest partner. What then? To truly believe it, to truly feel it, we have to bring that sense of love and compassion to ourselves. Only we are with us all the time.

Exercise

Try the same exercise again. Take a quiet minute and slowly repeat to yourself: 'may I be happy, may I be healthy, may I live with ease.' Allow yourself a few minutes just to feel those words as you repeat them.

The most fundamental aggression to ourselves, the most fundamental harm we can do to ourselves is to remain ignorant by not having the courage and the respect to look at ourselves honestly and gently.
Pema Chödrön, *When Things Fall Apart:*
Heart Advice for Difficult Times

So we must come back to our own being. Be gentle to ourselves. Be kind to ourselves. Show compassion to ourselves. Look at the words we use to describe ourselves, the thoughts we use to speak to ourselves, the actions we bring to ourselves. Are they honest and true, or are they aggressive and cruel? Can we bring the gentleness and kindness that we would bring to anyone else to ourselves?

Mindfulness is an active engagement in what we already have. It is an active pleasure-seeking in the people and places around us. It is light, benign and joyous. It is social, as it seeks out others, rather than focusing on negative thoughts and feelings inside us. It is an understanding that, as imperfect as any day may be, we are living it now and we should seek out the magic this moment might bring.

How Not to Be Unhappy

The Black Dog Barks

Everywhere life is full of heroism.

DESIDERATA

Winston Churchill often described his own depression as a black dog and this book is, in a sense, about taming your own inner black dog. Our brain is an extraordinary organ that 'creates' sound, vision, memories, thoughts, emotions, as well as controlling the whole mental world we inhabit. Throughout our lives these experiences (thoughts, emotions, memories) are, for the most part, happy or at least neutral. But for all of us, at some time or other, they may become negative. Because we are on the inside experiencing these emotions, it can be difficult to see it from the outside; sometimes we need help from someone else to help us face our problems objectively. I hope that this book will help you see them from the outside.

Our brains can create negative emotions and negative thoughts at any time in our lives, but especially during times of stress. We need to become active observers of our own mental health problems and look after them in the same way we do other aspects of health. We may say we do this already but the reality is only 25 per cent of us seek support for mental health difficulties when we experience them. What we actually do is say: '*I don't matter; other priorities are more important. I'll push through.*'

Depression affects about three hundred thousand people in Ireland today. The World Health Organisation (WHO) has suggested that depression has an adverse impact on the individual equivalent to that of Parkinson's Disease; however keep in mind that Parkinson's tends to strike when people are in their sixties. Depression, on the other hand, is most likely to arise when we are in our twenties. It can trap us in our own home, on our own couch, in our own bed. How can we fight it? In this chapter I am going to discuss Cognitive Behavioural Therapy (CBT) approaches to depression. CBT has the strongest research evidence of any psychological treatment for depression. It is the front line treatment in Britain's National Health Service, is recommended by the National Institute of Clinical Excellence (NICE) and is enshrined in UK government policy.

Although there are lots of ways of framing the discussion, I am going to focus on one small, greyish, wizard of a man: Stirling Moorey. He is still alive and working in London. For most of his professional life, Moorey has, as part of his work, treated people with terminal cancer and depression – people who are in the worst possible position most of us can imagine. The remarkable thing is that they are in the minority. Most people with terminal cancer don't get depressed; doesn't that seem strange to you? You might think that if you received such a bad prognosis, you would instantly become depressed, but in fact most people don't. They may get low, they may grieve, but they don't get struck by the overwhelming physical, psychological and emotional tidal wave that is depression. Moorey has spent his life working with people who do get struck by this double blow of cancer and depression. He believes that they should be able to live free of this weight that holds them down beneath the waves.

This signals something important about depression. It isn't normal. Not everyone gets depressed at some point in their life. Unlike sadness or grief, it isn't automatically part and parcel of life. In fact although depression is an extremely common illness, it affects less than 10 per cent of people. It has its own logic and its own way of working. Depression occurs when those negative feelings take on a mechanism of their own, so that they don't lift naturally. We aren't able to see the bright side or even neutral side: we just see the negative.

Throughout this chapter, we are going to discuss the model that Moorey has put forward to explain how the mechanics of depression work. This isn't the only way to think about depression, but it is based on a wealth of research and real-life experience working at the coalface of mental health. What's more, it naturally flows into what we need to do to combat depression. If it can work for people struggling with cancer, perhaps it can work for us too.

At the centre of the CBT understanding of depression lies long-standing negative beliefs about ourselves, other people or the future. These beliefs may have developed a long time ago, in our childhoods or in our early lives. They may have come from negative events that happened to us, such as emotional rejection, loss or trauma. These events lead us to believe that this is the only way the world works. If someone influential in our early life failed to love us, we learn to believe that we are not likeable or loveable. If something sudden and tragic took place, such as the death of a parent at a young age, we learn to believe that our loved ones might be taken from us at any time. If we lost our home at some point, we might become particularly concerned about safety and security. These beliefs are often unspoken. We might not even know them ourselves but they act silently and powerfully throughout our day-to-day lives.

Nobody's life is perfect. We all carry negative beliefs. When these beliefs are coupled with stressful experiences (losing our job, experiencing severe pressure at work, a relationship break-up), all these latent negative feelings become activated in a very strong way. The old beliefs become very present and powerful.

Our brain creates sixty-eight thousand thoughts a day; it's an engine for thought. Most of these are neutral. They are thoughts about whether it is going to rain or not, chores we need to do, or an overdue trip to the supermarket. We don't even notice we are having them. It is not like trying to fill in a crossword where we are actively engaged in the process. They operate automatically. When something negative happens and our underlying beliefs get activated, these negative thoughts flow automatically into our daily lives. Suddenly the thought about going to Tesco becomes negative: '*I won't be able to manage*'; '*It will be too much for me*'. What in theory is a straightforward undertaking morphs into something vastly more demanding, as our thoughts fill us with self-doubt: '*If I can't even go to Tesco, what use am I?*' Our thoughts become short and rigid and generalised. We start to see only the pessimistic side of every situation.

What emotions are going to arise when people are thinking in such a way? Well, they are going to feel down but they might also feel anxious and worried. They might feel guilty and ashamed. They might feel angry. Depression isn't just about sadness. It is about the overwhelming weight of all these emotions. It is about the interaction between them. The sadness leads to anxiety as we begin to worry that things will never change; this leads to guilt that we are letting others down, or shame in case others find out our weakness. It is a wave of emotion that spins people around and around so that they can struggle to catch breath.

We react to all of this just as anyone would: we withdraw. We do less of what we normally do. This can be protective for a short period. We've all had times in our lives when we need to pull back a bit and take a little time out. But doing so over a longer period reinforces the negative thoughts we have about ourselves. The activities that give us meaning or even a simple sense of pleasure are curtailed: playing five-a-side, going out for a coffee or reading a paper. When we cut back on such activities, we have a lot more time on our hands for negative thoughts to grow. We start to believe that we are not capable of participating in hobbies or pastimes that we were doing with ease a couple of weeks earlier. As a result those underlying beliefs of being weak or not good enough are now reinforced.

Social contact is so important to our happiness, yet this is often one of the first things we neglect when we experience a depressive episode. We may go to work but avoid interacting with colleagues as much as possible. We may go out for drinks with a group of friends but distance ourselves from the conversation taking place around us; as such, we are missing out on the bonding that is essential to our sense of well-being. Without that social contact, there is nothing to interrupt our flow of negative thoughts.

Rumination is the process of dwelling and mulling over negative aspects of our lives (I'll return to that in greater detail in the chapter, 'Don't Worry Be Happy'). We keep asking ourselves questions: '*What if …?*' or '*Should I have …?*' We play out negative scenarios again and again. This amplifies all our negative thoughts because nobody has ever ruminated and come up with a positive answer. They always come to the most catastrophic, worst-case scenario – 'We'll lose the house'; 'I'll lose my job'; 'My partner will leave me' – whether this is a real possibility or not. Does this improve our mood? Of course not, it drives it down and down.

People react to low mood with negative thinking, increased avoidance, increased isolation and more rumination. How else do people react? Well, often people will do something unhelpful. For each person, this might be different. People might consume too much alcohol (and when we are down, even a small amount of alcohol might be too much). They might take recreational drugs or painkillers or misuse prescription drugs like Valium. Some people overeat, some people undereat. These are all understandable reactions to feeling depressed. They are short-term ways of improving our mood. The difficulty comes with the longer-term effects. Alcohol can have a depressogenic effect on our mood; overeating can affect our self-esteem, body image and overall health. Short-term fixes are just that: short term.

Depression is a deeply physical experience. It feels like

The Six Cycles Maintenance Model[1]

ENVIRONMENT

1. Automatic negative thinking

6. Motivation and physical symptoms

2. Ruminations and self-attacking

DEPRESSION MODE

Negative view of self, world and future

5. Unhelpful behaviours

3. Mood/emotion

4. Withdrawal and avoidance

DEPRESSION

carrying a heavy weight, so much so that even a short walk from the back door to the end of the garden can be overwhelming. We can oversleep or be struck by insomnia. We can feel lethargic and weighed down, or we can have panic attacks as adrenalin courses through our bodies. All of these experiences can happen to us at various points, which makes doing even simple things harder. A walk to the shops is a big deal when it might lead to a panic attack. Reaching work on time might be impossible if we feel too tired to get out of the bed when the alarm goes off. Many people with depression talk about feeling as if they are walking around in a fog, or as if their head is wrapped in cotton wool. These are physical sensations that make everything harder: work, conversation, day-to-day interaction. We all know how inhibiting a flu can be, now multiply it by ten and don't think weeks, think months. Much of this book is concerned with psychology but anyone who has ever experienced depression will agree that it can be just as much a physical illness as a mental one.

The difficulty in experiencing these processes – negative automatic thoughts, rumination, isolation/avoidance, unhelpful behaviours – is that they have a significant psychological effect. Each symptom starts to feed into the next. The more I avoid, the more time I have to ruminate. The more negative my thoughts, the lower my mood. The lower my mood, the harder it is to be motivated and so on. People start to ask: 'What does it say about me?' The answers they come up with are seldom positive. They see themselves as weak, or the situation as hopeless; they see themselves as being trapped in a system they cannot escape nor deserve to escape. Depression operates like an engine, each part conspiring to lower a person's mood. This is why not being depressed is very different from being happy. Not being depressed is about breaking down the mechanics – only then are we free enough to build the life that is going to make us happy.

This is the negative cycle of depression. The more symptoms we experience the more self-critical we get, and the more hopeless we feel about our situation. This is why depression can often last as long as it does and why it can often take people a long time to come forward and seek support.

So how does anyone get out of it? Despite the stark picture I have painted above, the evidence suggests treatment for depression is very effective. The first thing to do is to slowly deconstruct the experience of depression, as it is simply too vast to comprehend in its entirety. Second, we must recognise that recovering from any health difficulty is a process and will only happen incrementally, following a succession of small steps. Third, we gently and compassionately start to take those steps.

NEGATIVE THINKING

The complexity of our thoughts is worth reflecting on in some detail as they have a huge effect on every aspect of our lives.

‣ Consider this word: '*holiday*'.
  - What comes to mind? Perhaps a sandy beach, perhaps the thought, '*I need one of those*'.
  - How about these words: '*the last day of the holiday*'?
  - What comes to mind now? Maybe a feeling of disappointment or regret.
‣ These thoughts colour our mood.

Now how about this picture:

I'd like you to see the old vase.

By priming you to see one thing you preclude the other. How about seeing two faces?

The thought changes what we see.

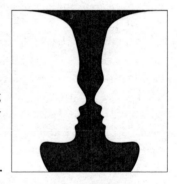

Now what do depressed thoughts do? If I have the thought 'I'm going to hate this party', I'm primed not to enjoy it; if I have the thought 'I'm going to mess this up', then I am likely to feel anxious, worried and stressed. The more negative the thoughts, the more negative the experience we are going to have.

What does it mean to have sixty-eight thousand thoughts a day? Do we think more than sixty thousand facts a day? Many of our thoughts are just opinions or whims with no basis in fact. You can think of your brain as a painter. Sometimes the thoughts will be realistic, photo-like recreations of the world around us but at other times they will be abstract, Picasso-like versions of events. It is important that we are able to sit back and notice the difference.

Begin by finding a pen and paper. Start to write down the negative thoughts that you have. Can you see the thought? Can you name it? Let's say I am going to go for a walk tomorrow. My brain tells me: 'It will be awful, I will meet loads of people I know. They will all ask how I'm doing, and why am I not in work? I will be humiliated.'

Notice that the negative thought wasn't *that* unrealistic. I might meet someone. It might be awkward. But also notice that it went a couple of steps past that. It was negative enough to stop me going. Maybe start to notice how unrealistic some of our depressive thoughts are. How *catastrophic*. And how neutral, basic and uneventful most of reality is. This is the dialogue we are trying to build up in our minds. Not rigid and catastrophic but flexible and realistic. '*It will probably be ok. I mightn't love it but I'll manage it'; 'If I re-engage with something I normally do, nothing catastrophic will happen. It might be boring or dull. It mightn't be perfect but it won't be catastrophic.*'

This isn't the end point of the journey – dull realism – but it is enough to get us moving. Happiness, the extraordinary wonder of being and the miracle of consciousness, are a few steps away. Let's get to realism first. I go for the walk. It lasts thirty minutes. It is not amazing. There is no extraordinary endorphin rush but nothing catastrophic happens.

There are five really common negative thoughts that people have:

- 'I'm not good enough'.
- 'If I try, I'll fail'.
- 'If people really knew me, they wouldn't like me'.
- 'Deep down, I'm not loveable'.
- 'I can't cope'.

Can you take note of those occasions when these thoughts occur? Write them down. Notice how frequent the thoughts are.

But also compare them with reality. Are they always true or are they actually only true some of the time? What have I managed over the last while? The next step is to go and test it out in reality. Let reality be the judge. If the thought is, *'I can't cope'*, let's see if that really is the case. If the thought is, *'I'm a terrible person'*, let's draw up a list of what we did today: got up; had breakfast; showered; went online; hung round the house. It might be short and it might be dull but there's little to indicate that you are a terrible person. Would you call someone else terrible for doing those mundane activities? The beliefs that we are trying to build up aren't ultra-positive. We are looking for realistic thought processes: *'I'll go on the walk. It will be ok.'* It won't be perfect but it won't be awful: *'I'm not terrible, I am good enough.'*

Often when we hit a speed bump, we stop. Our critical voice says we've failed, we are never going to get better, we are going to be like this forever – and we listen to it. Let's try to bring in a different voice, a compassionate voice. You mightn't realise you have this but you do. This is the voice you use when talking to a friend in trouble. When someone you love is worried or in difficulty, you always know what to say and are warm, open and compassionate. You mightn't know the answer but you know how to talk to someone you love. This is the voice we have to bring to ourselves. If your friend hits a speed bump you'd speak in an encouraging fashion: *'you are trying hard … you are doing your best … you are going to get there.'* However, often we bring a critical voice to our own activity. This doesn't motivate us. It just drives us down and down. With a critical voice, every speed bump becomes a full stop, rather than just a minor setback on our journey.

RUMINATION

Our brain is like a cow with an infinite appetite, not for grass but for the constant flow of thoughts our consciousness produces. Our brain likes nothing better than to chew these over and over. We can spend ours doing this. At its most pleasant, our brain daydreams. We can spend hours looking out a train window letting the world flow by and our thoughts drift pleasantly through the landscape. But at its most unpleasant our brain ruminates, it goes over and over anxious thoughts. It asks question after question: *'what if I failed my exams …?*; *'what if I can't get a job …?'*; *'what if my partner leaves me because of it?'* These thoughts always contain a grain of truth but we invariably gravitate towards the most extreme, worst-case scenario. We see catastrophe, followed by catastrophe, followed by catastrophe.

If submitting to pleasant thoughts is daydreaming then rumination is 'nightmaring': a constant flow of all that could go wrong. Except, unlike a nightmare, rumination doesn't last a few minutes but can continue for hours on end; so even small setbacks or issues can be magnified into major negative events.

It is not unusual to have a catastrophic thought or even to brood. I started driving again recently after years of living abroad where I didn't need a car. What sort of thoughts did I have: 'what if I crash?'; 'what if I can't drive properly and I block up a junction and drivers behind me start beeping?' All very normal. However, the key here is how long the rumination goes on for. If I think about crashing for a minute that will be negative. If I think about it for an hour, it is possibly paralysing. I might never get in the car, because my body is so anxious and my mind is so focused on the worst possible outcome.

So why do people do this awful, unpleasant activity? Because it can feel useful. We almost never ruminate on an insignificant topic. For me, I was worried about causing a serious accident. Surely that is a grave enough prospect that I should spend some time thinking about it? Surely I shouldn't rush into this? This logic is a *trap*. The answer to my driving conundrum isn't to think about it more. It won't make me a better driver. It won't make the roads safer. If I think that my skills are a bit rusty then I should book driving lessons, only drive on quiet roads, practise in car parks, bring an experienced driver with me and so on. I need to act, not to think. That is how I become a better driver, build my confidence and solve the problem. It is not a mental problem, it is a driving problem but as soon as I make it a mental problem, I am going to get trapped and paralysed by all the worst-case scenarios. If it is my honest belief that I am not a good enough driver at the moment, then I need to make a decision and stay off the road until I have improved. But if I believe that I can take a step forward then I need to do that, even if it provokes a sense of anxiety.

It is in this nexus that we see the interaction between anxiety and depression. I ruminate that something bad will happen, I become paralysed by it and then I start to believe that '*I will never be able to do this*'; '*I'm not strong enough*'; '*I'm not good enough*'; and I start to feel depressed.

AVOIDANCE AND ISOLATION

Much of what I have discussed so far concerns how we think when we are feeling low. But an equally important question is what do we do? This is generally an easy question to answer. Think of the worst hangover you have ever had. What did you do? If you are anything like me, you lay in bed, contemplated getting up but found it all too much. Plans were cancelled. Roles and responsibilities were pushed back to another time. If I had to be up and about then I felt like I was walking through the world with a couple of layers of gauze wrapped around me.

The most common behaviours when we are depressed involve isolation and avoidance. We see less of the people we normally see and we do less of the things we normally do. Many thoughts back this up: '*I couldn't cope with those guys at the moment; I'll only mess it up.*' These thoughts prompt a reduction in activity. And that is exactly what happens – our levels of activity go down and down.

One of the key aspects of depression is that it affects our capacity to enjoy everyday interactions or activities and so we avoid such scenarios. If we do stop, what fills the gap? Everything we talked about in the last section: rumination, catastrophic thinking, self-criticism, negative thoughts; if our mind isn't occupied, then it becomes filled with negative thinking. Our actions can help keep our thoughts at bay and a reduction in our actions allows the thoughts to rule the roost. So what can we do? The first thing is to identify what we do when we are feeling low. We will withdraw or avoid in different ways. Are there times and places when you feel worse? When are they? What is it about those situations that makes them so difficult? Notice the thoughts that those situations bring up. Is it at work, surrounded by deadlines and colleagues? Is it late at night, when there is nothing to focus on but negative thoughts? Is it early in the morning, when we have to get up to face the day? We may be in a room full of people but still find a way to isolate ourselves.

Often we notice that when we start to feel worse we become adept at avoiding normal day-to-day functions. We don't want to get out of bed. We don't want to go to work. This is where we have to go. We can do it gently. We can do it compassionately but that is the direction we have to move in. We don't have to do it perfectly. We don't have to be firing on all cylinders but we do have to do it.

No part of this will be easy. We may feel like we can't do it so we need to think small. Can we do half of it? Can we do 10 per cent of it? What is the smallest thing we *can* do?

Often when we're feeling low, the prospect of something as simple as making a phone call can seem daunting. Why not send a text? We mightn't have spoken to someone in a while, so send a short text by way of compromise. If we are struggling to leave our bed, begin by slowly bringing our two feet to the floor. We often say that depression is caused by the mind but solved by the feet. If we can put our two feet on the ground, can we then broach the possibility of having a shower? Don't think about it. Don't ask what comes next, just put your body in the shower. Afterwards get dressed, walk to the kitchen, put on the kettle, put a cup of tea in your body. For some people, at some times in their lives these are enormous steps. But nothing happens without them.

No matter what level we are at, these principles will guide us through:

‣ take small steps
‣ focus on the behaviour
‣ keep the focus away from the mind, and towards the issues or activities we have been avoiding
‣ keep it physical.

For some people, this might be getting out of bed, for others it is getting to work. For someone else it is getting the most out of the day.

When dealing with avoidance, the following patterns emerge:

‣ Depressed people criticise themselves for *only* getting out of bed or going to work. They compare themselves negatively to their well selves.
‣ Non-depressed people don't think about it at all.
‣ *We* are going to praise ourselves for the titanic effort it took to do it.

In many respects, athletes running marathons do not have to make the same kind of effort as someone with depression to go to work or to attend a social function. Depressed people are titans of willpower and we are going to *praise* that. We need to retrain our brains in order to celebrate our victories, however minor, and focus on our achievements. Today mightn't have been perfect; it mightn't have been everything we planned, but it was extraordinary and it is exactly the building block on which we can build a recovery. Every recovery is a citadel that we build brick by brick, and today we just placed another brick on the foundation. With every endeavour we undertake we need a cheerleader who will praise and encourage us, not only when things are going well but when we experience doubt or struggle. We are going to become our own cheerleaders.

We do not need to be cruel to ourselves to overcome avoidance. We do not need to be critical. We will not do this perfectly. On Monday, Tuesday and Wednesday we may be tackling these issues head-on but by Thursday we may fall back into old habits. That's alright. That's just human nature. Every diet and every new exercise regime anyone has ever tried has had these speed bumps and they are largely irrelevant. We don't even have to work out why they happened. We just have to roll onto the next day and go again. What was the plan? Let's get back to that.

We are going to tackle our avoidance. What else are we going to do? Let's do something nice. Before we had depression, what did we enjoy? We watched TV, we saw our friends, we went to football matches. These are the activities we want to reintroduce into our lives. Things that can bring us pleasure. They mightn't bring us immediate gratification, but they will in time. We just have to move in that direction.

We talked in an earlier chapter about the typical behaviours that bring us pleasure: food, exercise, sex, socialising, entertainment, giving, meaning. These are all good when enjoyed in moderation. These are the things we have always done and these are the things we need to embrace once again. What are the activities that once gave us a sense of accomplishment? There are lots of tasks that give a sense of pride when we complete them. Few people enjoy learning how to drive, but everyone experiences a great sense of accomplishment when they finally get their licence. There are many tasks that we don't derive much pleasure from, but the sense of accomplishment we feel when we see them through makes it worthwhile. We need to approach all these activities with a sense of balance. All things in moderation with nothing overemphasised.

'*I don't feel like doing these things.*' The worst part of depression – the reason why we get trapped by it and why we struggle to beat it ourselves – is that we don't feel like undertaking an activity, however simple it may appear to be. We know we should but we don't want to. It may sound counter-intuitive but often we *have* to do something before we *want* to do it. We take a walk, albeit reluctantly, and with time we discover that we actually want to do the walk. We go to social events, then we realise that after a number of occasions we begin to look forward to the outing. The old catchphrase, 'activation before motivation', is very apt: we do the action first and the desire for action follows.

If we think about it neurologically, it makes perfect sense. How do we know that we like cake? We try some only to discover that the body loves sugar and the reward system in our brain kicks in. The action comes first, the reward comes afterwards. With exercise we have to first confront the pain of stiff joints, and unpredictable Irish weather before the endorphins kick in and we feel a renewed sense of well-being. We have to make ourselves exercise before we get the reward for it, and then we want to build on that sense of achievement.

None of this comes naturally when we are feeling depressed but, like breathing through a blocked nose when we have a cold, it's really important that we keep doing it, however strange or unpleasant the sensation. Aim for small pleasures. Accomplish small tasks. Reward yourself afterwards.

CHALLENGE YOUR BELIEFS WITH BEHAVIOUR

We might believe: '*I'm useless at this. I'll never be able to do it.*' Something strange happens when we actually achieve that thing. We completely forget about it. We don't notice it at all. We don't recognise it. We just move onto the next activity we believe we can't do. We dismiss the good stuff and focus on the bad stuff. We shouldn't be surprised. Ignoring the good stuff is depression. One of the effects of this is that we never build up a sense of progress. We just have a sense of a series of tasks we feel we struggle to do, even if in reality we have already achieved a lot of them. We just focus on the next potentially 'negative' event.

I've discussed praising yourself after taking on a tough activity, but we can go a step further. We can examine whether the negative beliefs that we have are true or not. One of the exercises I ask people to do in therapy is to write down their attitude towards a certain activity, then to go out and do it. Afterwards, clients write down whether their fears were realised and, if not, to reassess their understanding of that activity. It's important to write it down because our depressed brain won't allow us to remember and focus on something positive or even neutral. In other words, we have to commit it to paper, otherwise our depressed brain will just dismiss it.

What should I write down? '*Went for walk. It was fine.*' Sounds stupid right? But it is vital because you need to go for a walk again tomorrow and you don't want to have to go through the whole thought process again. When it comes to tomorrow's walk you can try to balance the negative belief: '*I may meet someone while walking and find it difficult to chat; still, yesterday's walk was fine.*' This is how we progress. We build it up slowly and we remind ourselves of each small step we take. In a week's time, we'll be walking every day. We'll have a good exercise routine. Endorphins will kick in and we'll be in a better position to talk to someone if we do meet them.

For years people's depressive thoughts have been stopping them from doing what they wanted. By writing down the actual outcome of each event, we are using our own behaviour to challenge those negative thoughts. Our actions don't have to be perfect. They don't have to be back to normal. Writing down the positive things we do allows us to challenge those rigid, generalised thoughts.

Even a small behaviour can challenge a big thought. This is what I fondly term the 'Cornetto Principle'. One of the most corrosive negative beliefs we can have is that we don't deserve kindness. Let's challenge this. Let's buy a Cornetto. Just for you. For no other reason. You don't have to earn it. No one has to give it to you. By acting in a kind way towards ourselves, we can begin to challenge negative beliefs that we might have held for decades. Rather than try to talk our way out of it, we are much better off acting our way out of it. This small act of kindness allows us to challenge a long-term negative belief about our own 'deservedness'. Don't dismiss it. What would life be without small acts of kindness? We have to be kind to ourselves too.

But here's a couple of facts about the reality of improving our sense of self-worth:

‣ It will be gradual. All health comes back in stages.
‣ It will be mostly positive, but we can always turn a positive into a negative. We compare ourselves to someone we don't know (*they have a perfect life with no problems*), or compare ourselves now to when we were feeling great (*I remember coming to this pub and having the best night ever*).
‣ There will be some days that don't work.

None of these are reasons to stop. If we stop, we stay stuck. We have to keep going. Gradually, consistently, compassionately. People often ask is it worth it? No one can prove it to you in advance. No one can explain cake to you before you eat it. It will be worth it. Life is better than depression. It is a fact.

We always know what it means if we fail. It means we are a terrible person. We are a failure. It means we are never going to be able to achieve what we want. But what does it mean if we start doing these positive exercises? Often we just ignore it, or take it for granted. But if it is true for a negative event, it must also be true for a positive event. Maybe it means I'm an okay person; maybe it means I'm trying hard; maybe it means that

I'm a human that fails sometimes just like everyone else; maybe it means that as well as all the hardship, pleasure is possible too.

So where to begin? Let's start with what I want in my life. Most people don't look for something complicated. They want something simple. Let's start there. What would you like in your life in six months' time. A job? A relationship? Getting back to what you used to be doing? Ok. Let's pick the smallest step and start working towards it. What is stopping me: beliefs, worries, anxiety, low mood? Fine. Let's take that smallest step and see if we can gradually move towards that life. Let's gradually start challenging those beliefs with our own actions and the power of reality.

Depression affects our sleep, our energy, our brain function, our emotions, our thoughts. We wish more than anything that this would go away. That's not how health works. Good mental health inches its way back. Picture The Great Wall of China. Imagine the first step you take as you begin to walk along those ancient walls. Imagine with each step gaining strength and wisdom. Imagine with each step being able to look up from the ground and see the extraordinary splendour of China laid out in front of you. This is your journey. Breathe it in. Take the first step …

Did Woody Allen Have a Caveman Ancestor?

It did what all ads are supposed to do: create an anxiety, relievable by purchase.

DAVID FOSTER WALLACE

Every day, I hear stories suggesting that people are feeling more and more stressed. In day-to-day life, among friends, in the clinic, anxiety seems to be universal. Although we can often hear people being dismissive of anxiety – '*He's just stressed*', '*She's just a bit anxious*' – the fact is that anxiety can be hugely debilitating and a lifelong challenge. It's common and it's serious.

When the London School of Economics looked at the cost to the British Exchequer of anxiety disorders alone, they calculated that it amounted to some nine billion pounds per annum.[2] A crude calculation would put the cost to the Irish Department of Finance at seven hundred and fifty million euro per annum. This isn't small change. We could take 25 per cent of people out of the Universal Social Charge for that money. So it seems that if we can reduce anxiety, we should. We all know what anxiety feels like, but what is it, how does it work and how can we reduce it?

DIFFERENT TYPES OF ANXIETY

The first thing to understand about anxiety is that it is a very normal emotion. We don't want to experience too much anxiety or too frequently but it is a core part of who we are. There is no such thing as good emotions or bad emotions. Happiness and sadness, fear, disgust and shame are all part and parcel of being human. Anxiety is also part of that. When this normal emotion becomes overwhelming and occurs with increasing frequency it becomes an anxiety disorder. About 10 per cent of people will experience an anxiety disorder in their lifetime.

Emotions developed out of our evolutionary experience. The anxiety that we feel is about sixty thousand years old. We were programmed to feel anxious long before we were even born. If you can imagine how dangerous life was for our early ancestors you can appreciate why this was so. Humans were not at the top of the food chain and life was fraught with danger. We lived without electric light, heat or medicine. We experienced physical danger every day. One of our great adaptations is that we developed a shortcut to react appropriately. When we noticed bushes rustling, we didn't have to ponder whether the rustling might be dangerous or not because our bodies automatically sprung to action. Our heart rate and breathing increased. Blood was pushed to our hands and our feet. We were ready to battle or to flee: fight or flight. If a bird emerged from the bushes, our bodies readjusted accordingly; if a lion emerged, we were ready to run. Such a reaction had the potential to save lives and still does today, albeit in different circumstances. If your house goes on fire, you won't move slowly and mooch about, like you do on a normal day. You'll be up and out of the house faster than you ever thought you could.

So far so good, right? Here's the problem. In the modern world there isn't that much physical danger. Thankfully, we don't have to flee that many house fires. Most of the dangers that we face are emotional, social or personal. The situations that make us anxious take place in the family home or in the office; however, we are hardwired to behave as we would when confronted by physical danger and so we channel our inner Bruce Willis. We react the same way to an aggressive text as to an aggressive lion. I often use the analogy of a sensitive car alarm. Our body has an excellent alarm system but it can't tell the difference between a real danger (a car thief) and a false alarm (a football hitting the windshield). It reacts the same way regardless: adrenalin surges and we get ready to fight or run.

This has a whole host of consequences, but chief among them is that we can often have an overwhelming physical reaction to non-threatening situations. Our body will lurch into fifth gear but we'll merely be sitting in an office or walking through a supermarket. This is a deeply unpleasant experience. It is not dangerous. It is not harmful. But it is deeply unpleasant. We'll do anything to avoid it happening again, and that's where all the trouble starts: by trying so hard to avoid feeling anxious, we increase the occurrence of anxiety. This is known as the anxiety paradox. The more I avoid it, the worse it gets.

In this chapter, I am going to explain the CBT approach to anxiety. This is a highly effective, scientifically-validated approach to help us bring our anxiety response back to normal. Anyone can use it.

CBT has two important constituents where anxiety is concerned:

1. It asks us to go out into the world and find out whether our anxious beliefs are true. Is it a lion or a bird rustling in the bushes?

2. It asks us to learn to reduce our bodily reaction by gradually experiencing the anxiety. We train our body that supermarkets and office meetings are safe.

As I discussed in the chapter 'Change to the Power of Three', people will generally have a range of different reasons for experiencing significant anxiety: biological, psychological and social. Their feelings don't come from nowhere and some people experience anxiety for a very long time, perhaps for their whole lives. They may have experienced something in the past that makes them anxious now. It is real. It is physical. It is here right now. Why should they challenge it? People have to ask themselves: is their anxiety focused on that one trigger or has it become more pervasive? Is it affecting more and more of their lives? Are the things they are losing in terms of quality of life worth it? If we recognise that our own quality of life is being affected, it can be the motivation we need to begin change.

TRIGGERS

What triggers anxiety? Sadly, anything from impending driving tests to wedding days to speaking in public. Anxiety is a normal reaction to a new or challenging activity. We are anxious, as we should be, on the first day in school, a first date, the first day in work, the first steps into parenthood. But when one particular event becomes the focus of all our anxiety and consumes our thought process for days at a time, to the extent that anxiety significantly interferes with our functioning and our quality of life, we need to work on it. Often this is what we label an anxiety disorder.

Anxiety disorders take a variety of forms. Most people will be aware of panic attacks or Obsessive Compulsive Disorder (OCD) but few are familiar with health anxiety or social anxiety or Post-Traumatic Stress Disorder (PTSD), even though they are nearly as common.

A panic attack occurs when our anxiety levels suddenly peak – often without much warning – and we have an overwhelming feeling that something awful is going to happen to us. For some people this might be the fear of fainting or having a heart attack; for others, it is a vague sense of dread.

We often see OCD represented on films. Jack Nicholson needs to wash his hands one hundred times in the movie *As Good As It Gets*, for instance. In everyday life, OCD is less dramatic but often more overwhelming: an anxiety-provoking thought comes to mind and the person has to do something to make the thought go away. In our own small way, we have all had this experience. We are halfway down the driveway, when we wonder whether we have left the iron on or the door unlocked. However, instead of being able to ignore it, the anxiety is so overwhelming that we have to go back to check. But what happens if the thought occurs again and again? How many times are we going to check? Once, twice? What if the sense of anxiety actually grew every time we checked, until we had to repeat the activity one hundred times?

Everyone gets nervous when speaking in public but in the case of social anxiety all those common thoughts – *'I'm going to make a mistake'; 'they'll all hate me'; 'they'll notice my sweat and jitters'* – happen in nearly every social situation. Imagine experiencing the anxiety of a job interview every day, in every conversation, just sitting at your desk or in a lecture hall or on the bus.

PTSD happens when we have a permanent anxiety reaction after a traumatic event. Our body learns that something is dangerous: a sound, a smell, the feeling of being in a crowd. These can trigger the rush of anxiety and the memory of the trauma. In this way, people can struggle to get back into a car after an accident, or go back into a bank after being caught up in an armed robbery.

With health anxiety, we become highly anxious about the possibility that we may have a serious illness. In a vicious circle, the thought of having cancer, for instance, increases our feelings of anxiety, which generates physical symptoms that are then misinterpreted as cancer.

Generalised anxiety is when we can become very worried about anything and everything. I spend the chapter 'Don't Worry, Be Happy' dealing with it.

Although knowing what triggers our anxiety is important, it is not the key to making it go away. This is because other than avoiding our triggers, we often can't change them. We may have a phobia of spiders but we can't avoid all spiders. We may get anxious in crowds but we can't stop people congregating. We may become highly anxious about unpleasant thoughts but this does not reduce them or stop them coming. Identifying the trigger without dealing with the root cause often leads to worrying about it excessively. Avoidance and worry don't decrease anxiety, they ramp it up. So, although it is important to identify what triggers our anxiety, it is not the key to reducing it.

CBT Maintenance Model of Anxiety[3]

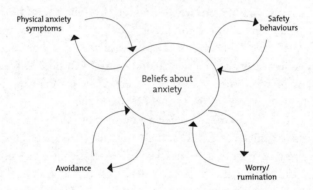

There are four key factors in maintaining our sense of anxiety. The more they come into play, the more our anxiety increases and vice versa. Ironically, often people's biggest anxiety doesn't derive from some external force but from the anxiety itself. The lifeblood for anxiety disorders is the fear of anxiety. As people put themselves into stressful situations, their anxiety increases. People then panic and worry about whether they can cope.

There's some important information to understand about anxiety. It is natural; it developed to keep us safe from threat; and, though it is highly uncomfortable to experience, it is not dangerous. Billions of people in the world will be anxious today. Some of them will have been anxious for decades. It is an awful feeling, but worrying about it only aggravates it further. One of the key lessons to teach ourselves is that anxiety, though deeply unpleasant, is not dangerous. We need to acknowledge to ourselves that worrying about our worry won't make us better. If you add up all the time you have spent worrying, it amounts to several thousand hours. If thinking could have got you out of this problem, it would have already. If you want to feel differently, you need to do something differently.

PHYSICAL ANXIETY

So what does our body do when we feel anxious? Well, it prepares for a 'fight or flight' scenario and so our heart rate, adrenalin levels and blood pressure all increase. This reaction has a couple of interesting side effects. People are often sitting or just standing still when it happens. The body is like a car revving. It is desperate to move but we are in the office or in a crowded shop and so have to stay where we are. This creates a desperately uncomfortable feeling. If we had the chance to go for a quick sprint or a decent walk, this feeling would quickly relieve the sense of discomfort, but we often don't have that opportunity. We can't leave the office every time we feel anxious. This emphasises the importance of regular exercise for people who experience anxiety. Just thirty minutes of moderate exercise daily will help burn off that adrenalin.

But how high is someone's heart rate when they become anxious? Surprisingly, not that high. In the department where I work, we have a staircase four flights high. A person experiencing anxiety will find their heart beating about as much as if they walked up those stairs. Anxiety feels so much more uncomfortable because it comes out of the blue; the person often doesn't know what triggered it, and their heart and lungs are moving but the major muscle groups are still. But your heart beats all the time. It is doing what it is meant to do. Your lungs work all the time. They are doing what they are meant to do. In fact, they are both working less hard than when you exercise. So the experience is uncomfortable but it is not dangerous. And that makes a lot of sense. The whole point of the fight or flight system is to protect us. If we keeled over every time we were startled by the rustling of a bush, humankind would have become extinct a long time ago. Our body is very good at regulating itself.

What are the other side effects?

‣ We often get a twitch in our hand or in a leg muscle. This is just the increased speed of our blood moving through the veins and muscles of our limbs, going where it is meant to go.

‣ Where does that blood come from? Well the blood is drawn from our stomach because you don't need to be digesting when you are running away from lions. This is what gives many children nausea on the first day of school. It's what makes us want to pee before big meetings.

‣ We also draw a little blood from our brain, because you don't need to be solving crosswords mid-sprint. This is what gives people the feeling of faintness or dizziness when they are anxious. However, it is important to note that it is impossible to faint from being anxious. Why? To faint your blood pressure needs to go down. When you are anxious, your blood pressure goes up. The one thing you won't do is faint (there is one exception to this, blood phobia/needle phobia).

‣ We feel sweaty, red-cheeked, hot.

All in all, it's a very unpleasant feeling, particularly when it blindsides us in front of witnesses. It's understandable then that these normal sensations can often be interpreted in the most catastrophic ways. A beating heart is interpreted as a heart attack; a flushed face is interpreted as something onlookers will mock; the feeling of nausea is interpreted as a serious, underlying illness; dizziness is interpreted as a sign you are about to faint. All of these normal sensations happen as a result of anxiety and, in a particularly vicious circle, conspire to make the anxiety worse.

What is the most natural thing to do in the world? Escape! But what happens if we don't escape? Exactly what has happened in hundreds of situations throughout our lives. What happened the second week after we started going to school? We became less anxious and started to enjoy it. What happened on the second date? We relaxed more and became more like ourselves. The fight or flight system is designed to give us a short burst of energy to get us out of a dangerous situation. It wants to regulate itself. If a person stays in the situation, the fight or flight response diminishes naturally. This takes about forty-five to sixty minutes. It is only if we escape that it suddenly resets itself and is ready to be anxious again moments later.

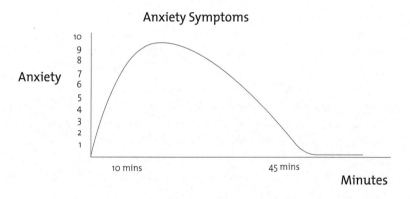

There is more good news. It is a learning system. The next time we encounter that trigger the response won't be quite so fraught. If we avoid, we teach ourselves that the situation is dangerous. If we tolerate the situation, we teach ourselves that it is safe. If we frequently return to the same trigger many times and stay until the response has gone down each time, the body will realise there is no danger and the fight or flight response will gradually go down itself.

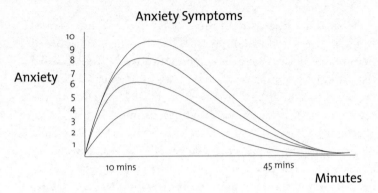

BELIEFS

I've been lucky in my life. I have only every had one panic attack – on the London tube the morning of New Year's Day; alcohol may have been a factor – but I had a mini panic attack quite recently. I had to have an MRI. I don't know if you have ever been in an MRI machine but it is a very enclosed space, very noisy and very restricting. Even knowing everything I know about anxiety, even having treated hundreds of people, my first thought was: '*this is very like a coffin. This must be what it's like to be dead.*' Do you think my anxiety went up or down? It went through the roof! It was only thanks to the soothing sounds of Lyric FM that I managed to stay in the scanner.

Think back to our caveman ancestor seeing the rustle in the bush. What actually makes him anxious? The noise, the sight of the leaves shaking or the belief that the rustling bush represents a significant danger? Our beliefs about the world around us have a significant affect on whether we will become anxious. Often our physical reaction is so quick that we don't notice that there was a quick-as-quicksilver thought in there too.

Anxious beliefs can be about different things. Here are some of the most common beliefs:

‣ Danger – '*I will get hurt*'
‣ Vulnerability – '*In certain situations, I'm powerless*'
‣ Embarrassment – '*If I do something, it will be humiliating*'

‣ Lack of control – '*I will collapse/faint/cry*'
‣ Physiological danger anxiety – '*If I get too anxious, I will faint/ have a heart attack, etc.*'

In fact, to really reduce anxiety, we need to work with the beliefs about anxiety. If our caveman friend believes that rustling bushes could be dangerous, he will always be wary of rustling bushes. It's not the noise or the colour. It is the underlying belief that associates these things with danger. He believes that a rustle equals a lion. To reduce our anxiety, we need to change the equation. Rustle equals bird. Although lions exist, it is probably safe to go into these bushes.

Often beliefs about anxiety don't simply plateau. They grow and grow over time. In fact, our caveman friend may become anxious of non-rustling bushes, shrubs and all sorts of benign undergrowth! If the belief is broadened, the anxiety will become more generalised. Our mind is powerful. It can imagine lots of dangerous scenarios. This is why anxiety doesn't stay still. It grows. People who were anxious about one thing ten years ago, can be anxious about one hundred things now.

With time this develops into an anxiety about anxiety. This is what stops people from doing the thing they want to do. If there is one belief that this chapter wants to address, it's this.

CBT encourages us to start looking at the thoughts that go with our anxiety and then judging if they are fair, reasonable and realistic. Do they apply all the time? Are they true for everyone? People with panic attacks often believe they might faint, but when you check with them they have often had hundreds of panic attacks but never once fainted. Something else must be going on other that fainting. What is it? We ask people to start analysing their beliefs about their own anxiety.

When we are anxious, there is a stream of thoughts going on beneath all our physical feelings: '*It's too busy in here*'; '*I'm feeling faint*'; '*I might collapse*'; '*It's too dirty*'; '*I might become sick.*' One simple way of reducing anxiety is to understand that a thought is not a fact. It's just a thought. Just because we think it doesn't make it true. How often, for instance, have we thought we couldn't cope but actually pulled through in a situation?

- We can challenge our anxious thoughts by recalling all the previous situations in which we survived.
- We can challenge our thoughts by writing down the counter-evidence.
- We can challenge our thoughts by finding balanced ways of looking at our experience. *'Sometimes I panic. It is awful but it won't make me faint.'*
- Best of all, we can challenge our thoughts by doing something different.

AVOIDANCE

Susan Jeffers' book *Feel The Fear and Do It Anyway* summarises a thousand theses in a brilliant title. Running away from fear seems like a sensible thing to do. Why would I do something that makes me feel uncomfortable? Tigers are dangerous; I don't walk over to pet them. But in the modern world our fears are more abstract and less straightforward. We fear judgement, rejection and serious illness. We can't leave these fears behind by running away from them. In fact the opposite happens: the more we avoid something the more it follows us.

Avoidance increases and perpetuates our anxiety. If we avoid something, whether it's the first day of school or a doctor's visit, it becomes harder the second time and even harder the third time. For someone with a phobia of social situations, speaking in a large group can create the same sense of anxiety our ancestors felt when they saw a tiger. But avoiding those situations will perpetuate that anxiety, not decrease it.

When we chart someone's anxiety over time, generally it increases over five to ten minutes. The person has a thought like '*I can't cope*' and then they remove themselves from the troubling situation. This makes sense. It is a pity it doesn't work.

By escaping, the anxiety comes down in the short term but the body learns that the situation is dangerous and the next time we are in the situation, we become anxious again. Not only that, the next time we think of or remember the situation we will also feel anxious. The anxiety grows.

This bring us to the Just Do It (JDI) principle. When we are anxious, we all notice the physical sensations: feeling sick or trembling hands. It is vital that we start challenging the anxious thoughts that go with these feelings. Equally, thinking alone won't get us there. We also have to 'just do' the thing and then do it again, so that our mind learns it is safe. If we experience anxiety, tolerate it and then go through the experience again, our body starts to acclimatise but we have also taught our mind that the experience is actually safe.

WORRY

It is very easy for people to get caught between worrying about stress and trying not to think about it. We can't tell our mind not to think about something – we have to tell our mind what we want it to think about. The best course of action is to engage with the environment around us: people, activity, work, pleasure. When we focus on worry, anxiety increases. When we focus on life, life increases.

SAFETY BEHAVIOURS

What are safety behaviours? Safety behaviours are small, subtle behaviours that we use to make the anxiety go away. We think they are making us safer but in fact they are reinforcing the belief that we are in danger.

Where are you sitting now? In a chair, in a house? Go lock all the doors. Turn on all the alarms. Barricade yourself into the room with all the furniture. Hold a poker in your hand. Do you feel safer or more anxious? The actual threat hasn't changed but by taking all these 'precautions', the level of anxiety you feel will increase.

Liz Lawlor, a well-known Irish psychologist, has elaborated on this idea. 'Before you go outside today, get an elephant gun. Shout really loudly, bang your feet. Walk all the way to the shops, shouting at the top of your lungs. There, it worked. No elephants will bother you today. This get-rid-of-elephant technique works every time'.

This is obviously a comic example. But we often do things in order to feel safe, even though there is no probable danger. We look for reassurance from loved ones. We check something multiple times. We look up the internet repeatedly to check for symptoms we don't even have. We get multiple appointments from doctors and specialists. We scan our bodies mentally. We scan our thoughts mentally. These things reduce our anxiety in the short term and perpetuate it in the long term. All of these behaviours will maintain your level of anxiety and won't decrease the realistic level of threat. We do it to feel safe but in fact it makes us feel unsafe.

We often think of these as 'just in time' behaviours. When you ask someone why he or she didn't die when they had their panic attack, they will often tell you that they sat down, 'just in time'. It was a near miss. Yet sitting down won't stop a heart attack. It might help you reduce your anxiety if you feel panicky but as a cure for heart attacks, no. These are the behaviours that allow all our catastrophic thoughts to thrive. I can believe that I just avoided becoming sick because I washed my hands for the hundredth time, or avoided a break-in by checking the doors were locked for the twentieth time, and so on. But this is simply not true.

Anxiety-provoking situations always feel like life and death. The situation always feels overwhelming, threatening and immediate. And I am asking you to go into these situations more often! In the beginning, people aren't going to feel confident doing something they haven't done before. But it is about treating it lightly. The anxiety will come – that's guaranteed. But notice it and get on with it. The more safety behaviours we use, the longer the experience will be difficult for.

THEORY A/THEORY B

How do we integrate all these different features of anxiety? The most straightforward way I have found is Theory A/Theory B.[4] We enter into the world every day with many different theories about how the day will pan out. We have a theory that rain will fall downwards (this theory is always proven correct). We also have theories about how our spouse will act (this theory is often proved incorrect). We have a theory about our anxiety. This is Theory A. This is any anxious belief that we have. For instance: *'If I go to a busy place, I'll collapse.'*

Other examples might be:

'If I go to out for a night, I might be attacked.'

'If I'm in a crowd, I'm weak and powerless.'

'If I go to the party, it will be humiliating and I will be rejected.'

'If I get too anxious I will faint/have a heart attack.'

'If I don't pay attention to this anxiety, then it will overwhelm me.'

'If I speak up, everyone will reject it.'

We live our lives as if this theory is true. We avoid lots of people. We stop doing activities. We seek reassurance from our loved ones that they will look after us. We check every situation we go into. We stop speaking up. We use avoidance and safety behaviours because we believe these beliefs are true. Safety behaviours and avoidance reinforce our beliefs about ourselves that we are not strong and that the world is a dangerous place to be in. We live as if Theory A is true. We live in a Theory A world. But we could live in a Theory B world. Theory B suggests that:

'If I go to a busy place, I will feel anxious but I won't collapse.'

'I may become anxious sometimes but I'll cope.'

'Most people don't notice when others speak, let alone reject someone because of it.'

'I can ignore my anxiety and nothing happens.'

Theory B is not positive thinking. It is realistic. We know we will feel anxious if we go somewhere busy but if we incorporate a realistic, rather than a catastrophic outcome, we'll be able to manage.

WHAT'S MY THEORY B?

If Theory B is true what should we do? Go to places, not seek reassurance, build up our resilience, reduce our fight or flight response.

When people are very anxious, they live in a Theory A world, but what if, in reality, Theory B was true? What if we were stronger than we thought and we didn't know it? What if the world was safer than we thought but we didn't know it? When we act as if Theory B is true, we reinforce the beliefs that we are more resilient than we thought and the world is not as dangerous as we thought; that we are better able to cope than we thought.

The goal of therapy and of this book is to get people to start testing out what it would be like to live in a Theory B world. You can't talk yourself into it. No one will be able to convince you. You have to go live it. You have to choose to go and then you'll find you are more capable than you ever believed, the world is better than you believed and the catastrophe doesn't happen. This is what it is like in a Theory B world.

How do you start? Begin by writing down all the experiences that contradict Theory A. This is not a diary of every time you have been anxious. You've been anxious a thousand times. But how many times have you felt anxious and survived? A lot, I bet. In fact, for someone with severe anxiety, they feel anxious every day, but they also survive every day. They may feel terrible but the catastrophe they are avoiding never happens.

WHEN HAVE I FELT ANXIOUS AND SURVIVED?

Now that you look back on that list, what do you notice? You might notice that you have felt anxious but still survived in many different situations. However, it is not enough to merely get evidence that Theory A isn't true, you need to get evidence that Theory B is true. Write down any experiences that show Theory B is true.

EVIDENCE FOR THEORY B BEING TRUE

You might have noticed that because we have been avoiding things for so long, we probably need some new evidence for Theory B. Where could you find some new evidence? What would you have to do?

- Do you need to go to the shops, speak at a meeting, leave the house without checking the locks, not spend hours worrying?
- Make a list of the easiest and hardest things to do.
- Start doing the easiest things.
- What happened? What did you learn? Write it down. Do I have any new evidence? What was good? What was bad?
- Let's look at a small instance of avoidance: what would it be like to drop one? How would that challenge Theory A and support Theory B?
- Let's look at some safety behaviours: what would it be like to drop one of those? How would that challenge Theory A and support Theory B?
- Let's start to play around with these behaviours and see what they tell us about the world we live in.

If you don't know where to start, try answering this question:

what would you like in your life? Most people don't want complicated things. They would like to see their friends more or have more free time or be able to embrace certain opportunities without feeling intimidated. In order to start getting evidence so you can take a Theory B approach, this is a good place to start. What would I like to do? If anxiety stops you from doing these things, then these should be the first targets to tackle. This way it isn't something random you have to do but something intrinsically rewarding. Start small. No one walks into a gym and picks up the heaviest weights.

Do one thing and see what happens. Was A or B true? Have a go at dropping an avoidance behaviour or a safety behaviour for a while. What does it tell you? Write down the outcome.

Now keep going. Keep doing the new behaviours and see whether Theory A or B is true. Keep doing your everyday behaviours and see whether Theory A or B is true.

› *'Went to the shops'* – Was Theory A or B true?
› *'Had a cup of coffee with friends'* – Was Theory A or B true?

By consistently checking our lives against Theory A and B, we can reassure ourselves about our anxiety and be in touch with the actual nature of world around us. Gradually, our belief in Theory A reduces and we can fully believe in Theory B.

This isn't a journey towards a fantasy but towards a grounded realistic vision. The Munster rugby team have a motto: 'you need the old dog for the hard road.' After everything you have been through, that's you. You are perfect for this road.

SELF-COMPASSION

It is hard work tackling anxiety. Most people try it and get exhausted by it and then stop. It is not that people don't try – they try really hard – but what's missing is the consistency. It is hard to keep going all the time. This is why it is really important to balance the hard work with self-compassion.

The ideas in this book are not another stick to beat yourself with. There is no point in sitting down at the end of the day and berating yourself: *'there's another thing I failed at.'* The point of testing something out is that you can't get it wrong. We are only hoping to learn from it. What did I learn by doing that today?

It is human nature to be inconsistent. How many of us have come up with New Year's resolutions in late December that are binned by the start of February? It's not just you; it is almost everyone. But we have to find a way that the work gets done anyway. The best way that I have found is focusing not on doing everything exactly to plan but on playing the long game. Know that every day won't be perfect; know that you won't always be hitting your targets and challenging your beliefs. The key is to not get disheartened but to come back gently and consistently tomorrow.

'I wanted to challenge myself today and I chickened out.'
Fine, no problem, what are we going to do tomorrow?

'I'd planned to go to the shops but it was just too much.'
No problem, let's go one step smaller the next time.

'I spoke up at a meeting and now I am a nervous wreck.'
Well done. Congratulate yourself for putting in such an effort.

'I went to town but came home having only completed half the tasks on my list.'
Excellent, that's more than you completed last week.

There is no point in focusing on what we didn't do. Just move on to the next thing we are going to do: a reward, a rest, a moment to praise ourselves, a gentleness towards ourselves, a smaller challenge. It's true for all of us. I didn't get that report written today – fine, I can only do it tomorrow. I have a long list of clients to see; ok, let's schedule some appointments and take each one as it comes. We have to bring some self-compassion to our work with anxiety. You won't be perfect. I won't be perfect. Fine. What can we do next? It doesn't matter if we only do a fraction of what we set out to do, as long as we keep doing it. We keep building. Every step we take is a forward step. Our momentum is much more important than our achievement.

Test out your anxiety ... then test it out again. But you need to bring a kindness to your efforts. You are working hard. You are making an extraordinary effort. Have a go living in a Theory B world. You'll discover something extraordinary. The world that you thought you were living in, the Theory A world, melts away to reveal the actual world around you. A world that is less threatening, less judgmental, less fearful than you thought. Day by day, begin to live in a Theory B world until eventually the old world you lived in becomes a distant shoreline.

Don't Worry, Be Happy

The mind is its own place and in itself can
make a heaven of hell, a hell of heaven.

JOHN MILTON

We all know what worry is but that doesn't make it easy to stop. Worry is daily; it is automatic. We don't have to learn how to do it. Even the happiest of us worry. We don't just worry for a minute. We can worry for hours, weeks, years. Ask a mum when she is going to stop worrying about her newborn baby. 2092? We all do it. Yet, study after study tells us that it interferes with our happiness. No other inbuilt mental process is so ruinous to our sense of well-being.

What is worry? Well, it is lots of things. It's mental: we can sense our mind thinking about something stressful. It is emotional: we can feel the unpleasant anxiety rising in us. It is physical: we can feel the knot in our stomach or the rising heartbeat. And it is repetitive: we can feel our mind going over and over the same issues.

The first thing to understand is that worry has a function. It is problem-solving for a problem that hasn't happened yet. We are not trying to figure out what our difficulties are but what our future difficulties might be. We can imagine that this must have been a very useful process for our early ancestors; thinking not just about how much food we have stored now, but how much we might need in the future, particularly if there may be a flood or a drought.

Being able to plan for the future, anticipate potential problems and solve them before they arise all seem like useful thought processes. So we can see why the caveman might have become a good worrier. We can even see why it feels so unpleasant. If worry was an emotionally neutral experience, like daydreaming, then we might never have been motivated to pick the extra berries or build the extra defences that we would have needed to ensure our survival. The unpleasantness of worry is a motivator towards action. I worry about berries. I feel awful. I pick berries. The worry goes away. I feel ok again.

So what is the issue? Pre-empting future problems and doing something about them in the here and now is a good idea. Worry without action just leaves us worried. Focusing on future problems without devising a plan of action is likely to leave us anxious and confused with no solution in sight. In fact, there comes a point when worry stops being a motivator and pushes us into avoidance and procrastination. We get so anxious about the problem that we don't even want to think about it, and we end up in an ever-escalating cycle of avoidance and worry.

Our caveman friend is worried about stockpiling berries for winter, but then he starts worrying about whether he will have collected enough: one pile, two piles, three? Maybe berries are the wrong food to be collecting. In fact, maybe instead of focusing on the berries, he should be focusing on meat ... What starts off as a reasonable worry escalates and pushes him away from useful action towards inaction. Ultimately he will have to make a decision: 'I'm collecting berries and three piles will suffice.' This may not be a perfect decision. He may not have got it right. But he has to make the best decision he can and then act. An imperfect decision is better than no decision at all.

The key difference between active worry and avoidant worry is being able to tolerate the uncertainty of the final decision we make. No answer we come up with will be the perfect answer and there may be some residual anxiety. We have to tolerate that anxiety and get on with whatever decision we make. This is where people become terribly stuck. They can't settle on a decision so their initial worry, which may have been useful, escalates and escalates until it becomes paralysing. People move from worrying about the most important things, to the most minor aspects of those things. Because the worry is now emotionally driven rather than realistically driven, people become focused on the most catastrophic outcome. Worrying about the least likely (the car crashing) and not focusing on the most likely (being late for crèche because of traffic), just leaves us even more confused than when we started. Worrying about the future so much that the present is zooming past us is a recipe for missing out on life.

I've never met anyone who says they would like to worry more. We are going to spend the rest of the chapter looking at how to worry less.

In psychology, we often use a technical term for worry: rumination. I dealt with it briefly in the chapter on depression. We use this word to separate out the everyday concept of worry from the clinical, technical and mental process. The word rumination comes from what cows do with grass. They chew the cud over and over, digesting it and redigesting it. This is what humans do with worries. We worry over and over and this can become a clinical problem.

Worry is a form of paying attention to our thoughts about past or potential problems. Notice that we are not paying attention to the outside world or to present events. We are paying attention to our thoughts about the past and the future. Hopefully, if we have learned anything from this book, it is that our thoughts are not facts. They are wonderful abstract paintings – some are soothing watercolours, others are filled with dramatic brush strokes – but they are not perfect representations of the world.

When we start to pay attention to our thoughts about things that could go wrong in the future, there is the potential that we spiral. We can worry about how we are going to finance a new car when the old car is working perfectly well; we can worry about getting sick when we are in perfectly good health. Worry is paying attention to our thoughts about future problems. So if we want to change our levels of worry we can change two things: how we pay attention and how we think about the future.

We will, because of our caveman heritage, physically react to worrisome thoughts as if they were true. If we think of cold on a sunny day, we can shiver. If we think of a plane crashing we can panic (even from the comfort of the armchair in our own livingroom). We know from extensive research that worry is directly linked to distress. The more you worry, the more distressed you become. If you halve the amount of time you worry, your experience of distress will come down. We don't expect worry to disappear. Worry will always be a facet of our lives but we don't need to worry as much as we do.

Worriers worry. They are almost professional at it. They worry when no one is looking. They even worry when they aren't aware of it. They'll worry before breakfast or while they are in the shower. Sometimes they think this is efficient but it simply distracts from the actual life they should be living, so obsessed are they with potential dangers and would-be hazards. They don't stop to smell the roses. They worry that there might be a bee lurking among the petals. People who are extreme worriers tend to worry for several *hours* a day. This ensures a level of physical anxiety bubbling away in the background and makes it easy for anxiety to become overwhelming. And people will tell you most of what they worry about is not important. They have simply gotten into the habit of worrying and don't know how to get out.

One of the key reasons people worry is because they are of the misguided belief that it's actually a positive in their lives:

'*I need to worry about the bills because I don't want to lose my house.*'

'I need to worry about my children because I love them and I don't want anything bad to happen to them.'

'I need to worry about the meeting next week because it is an important meeting.'

And these things are important. The question is whether it is useful to worry about them or not. We certainly need to act on them: pay the bills, ring the kids, prepare for the meeting. But is there any advantage to thinking about them for long periods of time? This is where we are mistaken.

People believe that because a particular issue is important, they should spend time thinking about it. Are you near a window? Go look at the sky. What colour is it? Blue-ish? That didn't take long. Now I would like you to spend the next ten hours looking at the sky. Do you think your answer would improve? In fact, your first answer, the one you made in half a second, is as good an answer as you are going to get and all you need to make a decision about what to wear. Mere time alone doesn't improve accuracy. We believe that it will but it is a false belief and it leads us into overthinking lots of events in our lives.

What do we overthink about? The events that have no clear answer. 'What will I do if I get fired?' 'I'll go on the dole; start looking for jobs; see if the bank will allow me a holiday from my mortgage; cut back expenses at home; try to get some part-time work from my brother-in-law.'

Now think about it for another ten hours. The answers you come up with won't be radically different. However, if you spend ten hours on it, you will be more anxious, you will have thought about a lot of catastrophic (*'what if we lose our home?'*) scenarios, you may even become paralysed and avoidant through anxiety. But you won't have a better answer. More time does not equal better outcomes, it just equals more worry.

Rumination Tree

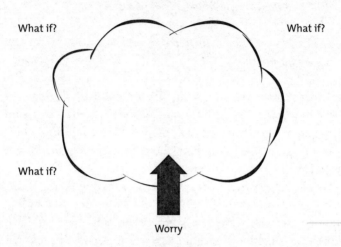

What if? What if?

What if?

Worry

Imagine an oak tree. A tree built of thought. Large branches, small branches, tiny shoots. Huge, ornate and majestic. Something that has taken years to grow. Now imagine it is rotten at its base. Every leaf at the top is pointless because of the flaw in its trunk. We build these extraordinary mental structures only for them to collapse on us.

The basis of this tree is the '*what if …?* What if this happens and what if that happens? We start with a genuine problem, then our brain starts to obsess over '*what if?*' scenarios and an hour later we are still circling the issue. We have thought about every potentially disastrous outcome – both likely and unlikely – without ever addressing the original problem. This is key for us to understand. Worrying about a problem takes us away from a solution. Worry is anti-solving. The problem is genuine. The problem is important. So we have to do something more constructive than simply worry about it.

Of course, people then behave in ways that exacerbate the worry and decrease the likelihood of the problem being resolved. Here are some typical examples:

- Seeking reassurance
- Seeking excessive amounts of information before making a decision
- Overlooking positive or neutral information
- Putting off making a decision/procrastinating
- Overanalysing problems
- Failing to delegate and taking on everything themselves
- Avoiding thinking about the problem
- Suppressing thoughts about the issue
- Becoming highly 'busy'
- Taking on different projects

Do you recognise any of these behaviours in yourself? If so, consider how they are likely to increase our anxiety rather than allowing us to make a decision and put the issue to bed.

Take the example of approaching the bank about receiving a loan.

- We can go talk to the bank and discuss options. The prospect of doing so is liable to provoke anxiety but, at the same time, is the only option that will give us solid information and move the problem along.
- We can seek reassurance from lots of people, but everyone we meet will give us slightly different information. How many people will we ask? Two? Ten? Not only is this a very time-consuming activity, we are unlikely to be fully satisfied at the end. In fact, we will probably need to go to the bank in any event.
- We can consult website after website and try to work out the best option for ourselves based on information from a host of banks. Apart from being an infuriating procedure, this will simply maintain those worrying thoughts.
- We don't think about the bank at all but we get worried every time an ad for a bank comes on the TV.

> ‣ We can say it doesn't matter and we won't make a decision but what happens next month when the overdue notice comes in?
> ‣ We can think and think and think and think and …

Ultimately, we need to find the best solution possible. We have to face our fears, manage our anxiety and call the bank. This is too important to worry about.

HOW TO STOP

Commit to worrying less

Most people readily agree to this. They hate their worry. They would love to worry less. But if you ask them to worry less about their children or their job, they struggle greatly. *'But my children are important'*; *'my job is important'*. We have to recognise that we worry about important stuff. Worry is just a useless response to something important. No one ever passed their Leaving Cert, got driving lessons, went out on a date, got a promotion, bought a house or kept their family safe by worrying about it. Worrying is something internal, private and passive. Any situation in the real world needs something external, public and active. I am going to return to this later, because of its importance; but for now we have to make a firm commitment to worry less. It achieves nothing.

Measure the problem

Worriers worry. They do it for many hours a day and they have been doing it for years. If worry was smoking, they would already be attending an oncologist. Because this has been going on for so long, it is an activity that has become automatic. Our first job is to begin to notice when we worry.

Although worry may happen at any time, people generally have key periods when they worry more. This might be early in the morning before the day begins or late at night when they have nothing to distract them but their thoughts. Equally, worry may occur at different points throughout the day. So take your phone diary (paper diary is perfectly fine too) and mark in with an asterisk every time and place you worry and a guess about how long you worried for (for example, 7 a.m.* *just after waking, for ten minutes*). This is important for two reasons. First, it makes us aware of a process that may have been automatic until now. We need to notice how frequently we worry and I think most people will be a little shocked at what they see. Second, we need to pinpoint those occasions when we worry the most because these are the times we are going to target.

After a week of measuring our behaviour, have a look at the pattern. When you total up all your worry time, how much is it a week? Five hours? Ten hours? Isn't that a little frightening? Think of what that does to your body. If we can agree that worry is going to prompt the release of adrenalin, then that's a lot of adrenalin. Is the last sentence kind of worrying? Sorry. Let's just agree that this is something we need to fix and agree that if you worried, let's say 50 per cent less than you currently do, that would be a good thing.

What else do you notice? Where do you most commonly worry? Is it in the car? In the kitchen? In bed? What times does this happen at? You are probably beginning to notice a key point about worry. It needs time and space. It happens when we are quiet, when we have a bit of time to ourselves. In fact, you may be noticing something else: worriers give worry time and space. They seek out quiet periods in their day or in their house, except they don't use it for rest or relaxation, they use that space to worry. Although they hate it, it is very common for worriers to believe worry is so important they make sure there is space for it in their day. Worry doesn't happen to you, worry is something you *do*.

Starve worry of time and space
Our long-term memory is amazing. We can remember tens of thousands of incidents from our childhood, but our attention span is quite short. A cognitive psychologist named George Miller discovered that our attention span is seven chunks of information, give or take two chunks. In other words, we can retain in and around seven pieces of information at one time. For instance, try to hold one mobile phone number in mind. Most people are able to do it. Now try to hold two ... Most people's attention span won't allow them to hold that much information. This tells us something vital about worry. If we give attention to worry, there is very little room to pay attention to anything else. We can be watching the TV and worrying, but we won't really be seeing what is on the screen. We can be at the dinner table but not really be engaged with what is being said. As a result, we are only half engaged with the world. This fact also gives us extraordinary hope. If we can shift our attention to the outside world, there is no attentional room to worry. The more we focus on the external, the less room we offer the internal.

If we want to reduce the amount we worry, we need to starve it of time and space. We need to look at those key times when we worry (because those will often be quiet, unstimulated times) and add extra levels of stimulation; we need to learn how to shift our attention from the internal to the external.

That doesn't mean we have to be busy 24/7. It means that when we want time to relax we fully engage in activities that are going to relax us. At other times, when we are quiet we need to be sure we don't drift into ourselves and stop engaging with the world around us.

The opposite of worry isn't withdrawal – it's engagement. So this process is about engaging with the outside world. What are the key times we have to target and how do we engage more during those times? Am I indoors, outdoors, in the car? The environment will determine what activity we engage in.

FLASHLIGHTS AND POLAR BEARS

When people worry they often get trapped in a bind. They worry about the anxiety it causes but they also feel unable to stop. Sadly, the human brain won't 'stop' thinking. It is like a flashlight. While we are awake, the flashlight is always pointed at something. We have to point the flashlight away from the worry and towards something else.

If I ask you to think of a pink polar bear, your brain is going to think of a pink polar bear. If I ask you not to think of a pink polar bear, then your brain is going to think of a pink polar bear. It can't help but focus on the object of the sentence. It doesn't even see the *not*. Golfers know this best. As you stand up on the tee, thinking 'don't put it in the rough on the left', there is only one place that ball is going. As all the best coaches will tell you, you have to visualise where you want the ball to go, not where you don't want it to go.

It is exactly the same with worry; we have to focus on where we want our mind to be. If we have decided that worry isn't useful and that it only takes us away from the real world, then the best thing we might do is decide to focus on the real world. Things that are external, specific, and here and now.

People can confuse this with distraction. We are not trying to distract ourselves from the worry, we are trying to engage in the real, concrete world around us – the world that really matters. If we are thinking about Miller and our limit of attention, we are trying to fill our attentional space with things that are going on in the world around us, not on the thoughts and feelings that are going on within us. If we are thinking about golf, we are trying to visualise where we want the ball to go, rather than picturing all the things that could go wrong. We are not trying to distract ourselves, we are trying to engage ourselves in our own lives.

Most people will recognise the times they are so busy that they do not worry. 'I had a million things on, loads of people were coming to the house. I didn't have time to worry.' This is what we are talking about, having people over and a full social life is a much better way to live than spending time alone with worry. Notice that when we are engaged in work, with friends, in a captivating movie, we don't worry. This isn't distraction, this is living. Notice that worry is the opposite of living. It occurs when we carve out time for it and devote time and space to it.

So here are some suggestions:

- Anxiety triggers the release of adrenalin, and exercise will help burn this off. Walk with classical music or a podcast on ear phones; walk with someone or with the dog rather than on your own.
- Listen to an engaging radio station, audiobook or podcast when you're in the kitchen.
- Have the radio on in the car.
- If you wake early and can't get back to sleep, get up, move, shower, breakfast.
- If worries creep in when you are exercising, increase the intensity of the exercise.
- Turn up the volume of the TV.
- Use relaxation tapes, guided meditations or classical music to relax.
- Go out for a cup of tea rather than staying in.
- If you find yourself drifting into worry while someone is in the house, engage them in conversation (really listen to what they are saying; really ask what is going on).
- If you find yourself worrying, get up, move, shift. Go to a different room, make a cup of tea, pick up a magazine, talk to someone, break the routine of drifting into worry.
- Send a text.
- Write an email.
- Read an article on your smartphone.
- Use your phone to take a photo of something that appeals to you.

So what have I got in my environment that I can focus on right now? Best of all is an activity: what am I going to *do*? Second best is something emotional or social that I can engage with. Third best is a solitary activity, reading/watching TV/listening to the radio/catching up with Facebook/writing the email you have been meaning to write/sending a text.

Obviously, we can't be busy 24/7. That wouldn't be healthy! So there is something important about learning the process of noticing when our thoughts have drifted inwards, gently and compassionately bringing them back to the outside world. Picture yourself at night, hiking along a forest trail. Your flashlight is focused on the path in front of you so that you don't lose your footing. Notice when the flashlight moves off the path in front of you and gently bring it back to the path you are on. This might happen a hundred times on a hike, but it is no problem, bring it back one hundred times.

If we have a schedule, like the one in 'An Apple a Day', then we always know what task we are moving on to next. We simply move onto the next thing we planned to do. We planned to watch a TV drama, great let's do it, but let's really focus. You planned to shower and go to work. Great let's do it, jump in the shower. Whatever is going on in my real life will be more important than the worries in my mind. Shift the flashlight from the unlikely (the car crashing) to the important (being late for a meeting).

SOLVING PROBLEMS

What about real problems? The world is full of real problems: mortgage arrears, the kids failing school, deadlines in work, the world being a dangerous place, surviving in an economic recession, managing illnesses. There is no shortage of difficult situations we have to face, and there is no point in avoiding these or procrastinating. These are serious problems so let's deal with them.

The ironic thing about worriers is that they are generally terrible problem-solvers. They may have major problems but they are frozen into inaction. So the problems never gets dealt with. They think about problems. They talk about problems. They just don't do anything about them. They are like the world's worst politicians. 'We recognise that there is a problem and we are going to prepare a committee report on it. This will take two years.' All talk, no action. The lifeblood of worry is procrastination. We put off actions for days or weeks and this space is filled with worry.

Developing the art of decision-making is paramount in combating worry. The first thing to do is pick up a pen and paper. Don't try to problem-solve mentally. If you are a worrier, this is going to quickly spin off into space. Using a pen and paper …

‣ Write down the problem or the question.
‣ Now write down every solution you can think of.
‣ Now write down the first action you can take for each solution.
‣ (Maybe you need to do a pros and cons list.)
‣ Pick the best option.
‣ Do the action. Now.

Some solutions will be obvious; others less so. Make your best guess. The amazing part of writing things out is that it clarifies the question, simplifies your options and reduces the number of possible actions. It discards the improbable, worst-case scenarios, allowing us to focus on the most realistic. Often the best option emerges from the process. Let's take some examples:

Should I go to the party?
‣ Yes – call and RSVP
‣ No – call and cancel
‣ Maybe – send a text to say you are not sure and you'll get back to them, mentally park until Saturday

I'm feeling sick. What should I do?
‣ Go to the GP
‣ Ignore since I know it's not too serious
‣ Give it twelve hours and see if it's still there. Meanwhile look after myself

I don't have enough money to pay my mortgage this month
‣ Mortgage holiday – ring bank
‣ Get loan – ring parents
‣ Sell house – ring estate agent

These are all real problems. They all need real solutions and shouldn't be ignored. In every case, there is a decision that needs to lead to an action. The key now is to take the action. Sometimes you will consider all three options because they are immediate, medium-term and long-term solutions. The important thing is that you are weighing up solutions, not simply catastrophising: 'What if the bank says no and then we all end up homeless?' Ring the bank. Find out. Then look at what the options are.

It sounds childish but one way of moving away from mental space (thinking) and towards the concrete and the practical is by writing down problems and potential solutions. If we stay in our minds, we are asking for worry to take over.

Decision-making generally involves three options: yes/no/middle option. The middle option is important because sometimes we have to find the halfway point, and this is the option we may have ignored. Should I exercise with my damaged shoulder: yes/no/gentle exercise focused on the rest of the body? If I get lost in extremes or catastrophic thinking, I miss out on the best option.

Let's practise it:

Decision Tree

What's the
question?

What are
the possible
answers?

What are the
actions?

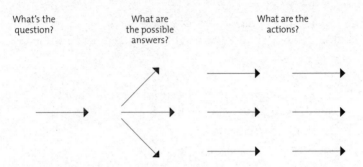

At the end of all decisions, there is a fourth option. Park it. Stop thinking about it for a while. No matter what you choose, you then have to decide to leave it at that. Park it. The easiest way to do this is to set a time when you are going to come back and review your decision. I am going to go to the party but I am going to review that decision at 4 p.m. on Friday. Then we use all the techniques in this chapter to get to Friday afternoon.

You would be surprised by the barrier that most people find to problem-solving like this. It solves their problems too quickly. They become uncomfortable with the idea that they can address a whole problem and come up with solutions with a pen and paper in ten minutes or so. Underlying the belief system of many worriers is the idea that worry is a positive thing to do. It prevents harm, or it is necessary to stop something terrible happening. When they solve a problem quickly they become nervous because surely it should take longer than that. They believe that the size of the problem should be matched by the length of time they spend thinking about it. This is not true! We can understand and solve lots of problems efficiently. Adding more time adds to greater confusion, less clarity and ultimately a failure to act.

When each problem is boiled down to three or four options, it creates a difficulty for worriers. They don't know which one will work. They want to be certain. They really struggle to tolerate uncertainty. It makes them anxious. So should they do A, B or C? And we don't know. Nobody knows. This uncertainty pushes worriers into doing all the negative behaviours that we discussed to try to create certainty. Except, as we have seen, these behaviours don't create certainty, they create more uncertainty. How can we know what we should do? There is a simple answer to this. We can't. Part of being human is not knowing the future. We don't know the right thing to do. Not me. Not the neighbours. Not our friends. None of us knows what to do. We know it is important not to do nothing. We know it is important not to spend our lives being anxious. But we don't have certainty about the right thing to do. The terrifying truth for worriers is that we have to make our best guess. This challenges lots of anxious beliefs that worriers have: '*I should never make a mistake*'; '*if I make a mistake, it will be catastrophic*'; '*if I make a mistake, it will hurt the people I love*'; '*it is better to be safe than sorry*'. We can see from our history how we might have developed beliefs like these. If something negative happened in our past, we worry that something negative will happen in our future. Worriers believe these thoughts so much that the prospect of making a decision – and possibly making a mistake – becomes intolerable to handle. What do non-worriers believe? '*I'll do the best I can*'; '*we'll muddle through*'; '*I'll tackle each problem as it comes along*'; '*life works out*'; '*you can only do what you can do*'. There are two distinct philosophies here. Non-worriers don't have more certainty about life's problems, they just tolerate the uncertainty better. They do that using beliefs like those above. Your job is to go out into the real world and test out which philosophy is more realistic. You can do this gradually, gently and compassionately but always moving towards greater toleration of the uncertain.

I am not suggesting that life is perfect or that bad things never happen. But I am suggesting that life is considerably easier than the worries our mind allows us to see. But don't listen to me. Go out and see. Make a decision quickly. See what happens. Don't look for advice or reassurance. See what happens. If you start to notice that, actually, we are able to muddle through and figure things out as we go along then you are closer to being a content human in a stressful world.

Surfing the Wave

Emotions in my experience aren't covered by single words ...
I would like to have at my disposal complicated hybrid emotions ...
like say, 'the happiness that attends disaster' or 'the disappointment
of sleeping with one's fantasy' ... I would like to have words for 'the
sadness inspired by failing restaurants' as well as for 'the excitement
of getting a room with a mini-bar'. I've never had the right words
to describe my life and now that I have entered my story I need
them more than ever.

JEFFREY EUGENIDES

Let's think about our emotions for a while. We recognise that we all have emotions, all the time. Think of them like a pulse beating in the background. We generally don't notice them unless something dramatic happens and we feel a surge of happiness or sadness. Our emotional life tends to regulate itself: gently up and down. Generally, we don't feel as upbeat on Monday mornings as we do on Friday afternoons. When good things happen we get a lift; when bad things happen our mood drops. Our moods don't change radically day-to-day or hour-to-hour. Like a pulse, they rise and fall.

We also recognise that our friends and families have very different emotional lives. Some people are more emotional than others. We will have friends who seem to thrive on drama and others who are rarely fazed. There is nothing intrinsically right or wrong here, it is just the wonder of life. Variation is the norm. Often we see this echoed in the national stereotypes we use.

These are gross generalisations but they are a useful shorthand to describe different ways of experiencing emotion. We consider the clichéd German as solid, steady and in control. We see the clichéd Spaniard as hot-headed, passionate and prone to gesticulation. This is wonderful. It is part of the joy of living. We enjoy having the company of both types of people for different reasons.

Emotional dysregulation is probably a term that most people are not familiar with. It refers to being frequently overwhelmed by emotions. The person doesn't just feel low or anxious. They feel low, anxious, angry, embarrassed, guilty, ashamed, all at once. This can happen very rapidly, out of the blue. Someone can feel fine in the morning and hugely upset an hour later. This creates the feeling of emotional overload which is unpleasant, unpredictable and distressing in itself.

Emotional dysregulation is most commonly associated with the diagnosis of Borderline Personality Disorder (BPD). While this disorder is rare we have found that emotional dysregulation crops up for a wide number of people in the population with a whole range of mental health difficulties like anxiety and depression. There is a growing body of research with similar findings. Researchers have found that around 14 per cent of the general population has regular experiences of emotional dysregulation. This does not indicate a problem per se, but does raise their risk of other mental health issues. Because being regularly emotionally overwhelmed is unpleasant and difficult to deal with, it can often lead to becoming anxious, or feeling depressed or attempting to self-medicate with alcohol or disordered eating. It doesn't cause any of these mental health difficulties but can increase the risk of developing them and can interfere with recovery from them. For instance, emotional dysregulation has been associated with eating disorders, depression, anxiety disorders, substance use disorder and attention deficit disorder. So it is fair to say that emotional dysregulation is common across the population and occurs alongside a lot of other difficulties.

I find that I meet lots of clients with anxiety and depression who also have difficulties with emotional dysregulation, and that it is necessary to address this in order to tackle the anxiety and depression. While the level of emotional dysregulation would not be of the severity to lead to a BPD diagnosis, it is a significant factor in keeping the anxiety or depression going.

UNDERSTANDING EMOTIONS

How is emotional dysregulation different from, say, depression? When people become depressed, their mood drops consistently over a significant period of time, be it weeks or months. They may feel a variety of negative emotions (e.g. anxiety or guilt) but the primary sensation is one of low mood. With emotional dysregulation, someone's mood bounces up and down. They may feel brilliant in the morning, terrible in the afternoon and brilliant in the evening again. The constant shift in mood becomes very difficult to manage. It isn't typified by one single emotion but a whole wave of emotions crashing over the person so that they can struggle to pick themselves back up again.

Emotional dysregulation is often misunderstood. This is because its nature is essentially changeable. Unlike other mental health problems which stay fairly static, emotional dysregulation changes all the time. If someone is depressed today, chances are they are probably going to be fairly depressed tomorrow. If someone is anxious about socialising today, they are most likely to feel anxious about socialising tomorrow. But this is not the case with emotional dysregulation. It bounces around. I can feel low and depressed today but be bustling with energy tomorrow. I can have panic attacks the day after that. This is infuriating for the individual and can be difficult for friends and family to understand. Equally, people with emotional dysregulation can behave in different ways. Some will struggle with self-harm or addiction, others with romantic relationships or exams. The range of different ways emotional dysregulation can manifest itself means it is difficult to identify and to work on.

Emotions are neither positive nor negative. They are a part of being human. We are all built to feel happiness, sadness, fear, worry, embarrassment, guilt. They are as much a part of us as our fingers and toes. We can't avoid sadness any more than we can be constantly happy. We are simply not built like that. We can try to suppress emotions but they pop back up. We can suppress our frustration at our boss but it erupts later in an argument with our partner or in a display of aggression towards another driver on the commute home. The emotion has a life of its own.

When we talk about emotion, it is easy to blame ourselves. What is a 'normal' amount of emotion? Earlier we talked about the Spanish and the Germans. This is a gross generalisation but it serves its purpose. The norm is different for different people. Some people are 'Spanish' and some people are 'German'. More often, difficulties arise when a 'Spaniard' is born in a 'German' household. Everyone else operates without any fuss. Never any tears. Never any bursts of excitement. They can't understand this strange nationality in their midst. This person filled with whoops of laughter and moments of distress. By either accident or design, the person gets the message; *why can't you feel less?* You might as well ask a leopard to change its spots. Often the Spaniard starts to pretend, starts to suppress, starts to worry, starts to see their normal emotions as something pathological, something alien to be fought. They try to make the emotions go away: by ignoring them, by drowning them in alcohol or food, sometimes by self-harming. All of these reactions make sense. They just won't work. The emotions will always win out. The emotions will emerge, a storm on the horizon.

All emotions developed during our evolution. They carry the ability to spark us into action. Negative emotions have a function. Anger makes us ready to attack. Fear makes us ready to escape. Sadness pushes us to withdraw from hurtful situations. If we didn't experience negative emotions, as a species we would not have made it this far. However, we can become 'phobic' of our emotions. We hate being at the mercy of our emotions and would like to be in control at all times. Yet, sixty thousand years of evolution are going to override our desire to pretend that something isn't bothering us. This can work for a while but, ultimately, it is destined to fail. So if we suppress our emotions, they are going to bounce back. Evolution will win out.

Emotional dysregulation occurs when our emotions take over and we become overwhelmed. This often occurs rapidly and changes hour-by-hour or day-by-day. People often describe this as very distressing. It is not a problem if it happens every now and again – this is very normal. But if it happens all the time, people can struggle to manage it and often use extreme or addictive behaviour as a coping mechanism. When people resort to extreme or addictive behaviour, the cure is often worse than the problem. Emotional dysregulation is an experience of extremes: extreme emotion, extreme behaviour and extreme thoughts.

The problematic behaviours arise:

▸ either as a natural consequence of intense emotions. So, for instance, I shout at someone because I'm angry;

▸ or as an attempt by the person to regulate their own emotion. So, for instance, I use alcohol to reduce anxiety or totally withdraw from everyone to feel less frustrated.

These behaviours reduce the emotions in the short term, but cause greater harm in the long term. When someone is hit by a wave of emotion, they have more extreme thoughts than normal. They might believe that '*I can't cope*'; '*everything is too much*'; '*I'm useless*'; '*why can everyone else manage?*'; '*I'm letting everyone else down*'. Do people feel better after having thoughts like these or worse? Thoughts like these drive more distress, more anxiety, create a lower mood and are more likely to leave the person feeling dismayed. However, there is a middle ground between feeling nothing and being overwhelmed. In order to live with our emotions, we have to have a mindset that incorporates them into our lives. I am emotional. I will be emotional at times. I need to be accepting of this. But what are the forms of behaviour that are helpful to me so that I don't become more distressed than I can deal with and so that I can enjoy life to the full?

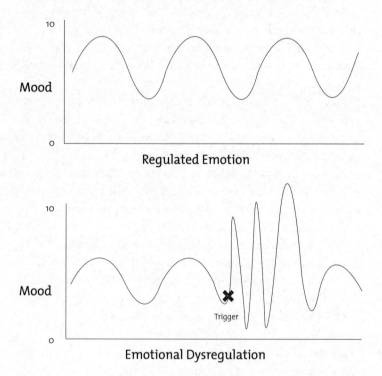

Regulated Emotion

Emotional Dysregulation

We need to know who we are, then we can really work the way we want to. But that doesn't mean we want to be overwhelmed by our emotions all the time. Every chapter in this book is relevant to emotional dysregulation and generally we can use them all.

A BALANCED LIFE

The best place to start is by understanding and accepting our emotional lives. We are going to be emotional people but how do we react to this? Often people with emotional dysregulation have quite dysregulated behaviour. They are either overbusy, not engaged at all, or flipping between the two. What we are going to strive for is balance. Not perfection. Not all the time. Just to live relatively balanced lives as best we can.

As each of us experiences emotion differently, we will each have different patterns of distress. We can begin to examine the thoughts and behaviours that exacerbate and maintain the extreme emotion. Initially we look to reduce any extremes of behaviour. Do we work too much? Lie in bed too much? Drink too much? People are often very aware of these behaviours but have struggled over a long period to do anything about them. It is very common to see someone with extremes of emotion react with extremes of behaviour. These behaviours perpetuate and maintain the emotion, so if we want to reduce the 'strength' of the emotion, we can begin by reducing the 'strength' of the behaviour.

The next step is to take the middle ground. The first thing we ask people to do is draw up an activity schedule (on the next page) and start to plan out their week. Where does the work go? Where does the exercise go? Where does the socialising go? As we saw in 'An Apple a Day', we need to incorporate all of theses aspects into our lives in order to be happy. Often emotional dysregulation pushes them out of our lives. We need to start putting in all of these areas of balance: time alone/time with people; time to rest/time to be active; time for pleasure/ time for work; time to eat/time to sleep.

It is amazing how often people with emotional dysregulation have schedules that three people couldn't achieve. The constant busyness is a way of avoiding the emotion, but like all maladaptive behaviours it doesn't work. We become exhausted. We become cranky. We become ill. We get annoyed that we

	MORNING	AFTERNOON	EVENING
MON			
TUE			
WED			
THUR			
FRI			
SAT			
SUN			

are unappreciated. Busyness is not a replacement for balance. So there is something important about slowing down, being realistic, saying no to something. Look at the schedule. Keep asking yourself: where is the balance?

It is very hard to stop a behaviour. It is much easier to replace a behaviour. When and where do my more extreme behaviours happen? People might drink too much on a Saturday night, meaning they feel particularly emotional on Sundays. If we want to reduce the amount we drink on Saturday night what are we going to do instead? Go out to dinner instead of the pub? Arrive an hour later than we normally do and get the last bus home rather than an early-morning taxi? What moderate behaviour are we going to use to replace our extremes of behaviour?

If I can never get up for my first lecture on Mondays, what is happening on Sunday evenings that might be aggravating the problem? Am I worried? Am I handing assignments in late and becoming very anxious about attending classes as a result? In order to reduce the extreme behaviour, generally we have to look at the balance across the whole week and replace the maladaptive behaviour with something more moderate. If I can never get my work in on time, I need a gentler, more consistent schedule during the week. If I am overcome by worry on Sunday nights, can I try to distract myself by watching a light-hearted movie or reading a chapter of a good book?

It is extraordinary how physically run down people with emotional dysregulation generally become. The chapter 'Get the Body Right' is really important here. We have to be physically balanced to feel emotionally well. Rest, exercise, food. A lack of these will trigger emotional overwhelm, while ensuring all these are in balance will calm us. So get the schedule out. Where are rest, exercise and food going to go? Am I making time for lunch? Am I eating enough? Am I taking enough breaks, enjoying myself?

I was recently talking to someone who decided to begin eating well by adopting an all-juice diet with extra wheatgrass shots. Unsurprisingly, it didn't work so well. The diet proved too extreme, difficult to sustain and lacking in pleasure. The person's mood was all over the place. We need to eat healthily of course, but should do so with a sense of balance.

Emotional suppression

The one thing you can't do when we are in the middle of a storm is pretend the storm doesn't exist. If you pretend a storm isn't there, you end up very wet indeed. You can choose any middle-way behaviour you like to manage it – stay at home; wear waterproofs; bring an umbrella – but you can't pretend it doesn't exist. Yet this is exactly what we often do.

Because we are Spanish in a German world, we pretend to be German. We pretend we don't feel annoyed when we really are. We pretend we are happy when we are really upset. We pretend that we aren't worried when we actually are. Emotions are akin to boomerangs: the further we throw them, no matter how far you throw them they always come back. For people with emotional dysregulation, they often try to throw them very far away indeed. This only means the emotion comes back at full force.

We have to accept that we are emotional and we have an emotion right now. It is not a catastrophe. It is not a personal failing. It is just who we are and the situation we are in today. After that we can do whatever we like. Any middle path behaviour will be beneficial. We want to stay home for a day. Fine – as long as we don't stay home for ten consecutive days. We want to exercise. Fine – as long as we don't work out so much that we injure ourselves. Clean the house. See our friends. Take a break. All of these activities are good and beneficial as long as we don't take them to an extreme. Yet the pattern is often to suppress, suppress, suppress, feel overwhelmed and then extreme, extreme, extreme behaviour in order to numb out the emotional distress.

RUMINATION

People with emotional dysregulation often have a high level of rumination. They become overwhelmed, withdraw and dwell on all the factors that caused the overwhelm. This is really unhelpful and prolongs their distress. The chapter 'Don't Worry, Be Happy' has lots of techniques on reducing rumination, if someone does withdraw because they feel overwhelmed.

CATASTROPHISING SITUATIONS

Extremes of emotion can lead to extremes of thinking. A problem is never just a problem – it is a catastrophe. Small things are seen as big things. This feeds back into our emotions. We feel more anxious, more distressed, more worried when we are dealing with a potential catastrophe than when we are dealing with an everyday problem. There is a significant emotional impact from catastrophic thinking.

If we think in an extreme way, we often act in an extreme way. If I believe the boss hates me, then I might quit in a fit of pique; I might drop out of college because I believe that I am not good enough; I might break up with someone because I feel that they are not loving enough. If I started to see these things in a middle way and started to believe these things in a middle way – *'my boss is cranky but doesn't hate me'*; *'college can be difficult but I can make it through'*; *'my partner is sometimes thoughtless but does love me'* – then I can manage them.

People often get caught between two extremes: *'I have to be perfect or I'm a failure'*; *'I have to get the promotion or I'll quit'*; *'If someone doesn't love me, they hate me.'* This doesn't mean people are wrong. There may be a problem. There may be something to deal with, but catastrophising doesn't help.

Come back to the middle way. What lies between these two extremes?: *'I'm going to make mistakes sometimes but generally I do a good job'*; *'If I don't get the promotion, I can look for another job but there is no rush*'; '*the relationship isn't where I would like it to be but I can see how it will develop*'. As soon as we can see the middle way, we can start to feel our emotional temperature drop.

Notice that we are not telling ourselves that everything is perfect. This is the real world; everything isn't perfect. We are looking for something realistic: '*I messed that up but it will be ok.*' When we are thinking of other people that set us off can we take this middle-way approach as well? '*My sister is a pain sometimes, but I love her and want to get on with her.*' This person is not seen as an angel or the devil, rather as someone human that we have a relationship with and have to figure out how to live with.

CATASTROPHISING EMOTIONS

A key part of this is that people often see their own emotion as a catastrophe. They feel that if they become emotional they will 'collapse' or 'won't be able to cope'. They see their emotions as something dangerous that has to be managed, suppressed or avoided. The chapter 'Mindful Living' is important here. Our emotions can be distressing. They can even be overwhelming. They are like the weather in so far as small winds can become extraordinary hurricanes. But like the weather all emotions pass. Whatever we feel now, we won't feel in a few days from now. Our experiences are essentially transient. So, although it may be highly distressing to experience overwhelming emotion now, it will pass. This isn't unusual. Transience is the norm.

Often people can think that they are their feelings. Imagine being a lighthouse keeper at the end of a long headland. The lighthouse might be buffeted by the storm. The storm might worry the lighthouse keeper, keep him awake at night. But night will pass, dawn will come, the sea will calm and the sun will rise. Our thoughts are not who we are. Our behaviours are not who we are. Our emotions are not who we are. We are the lighthouse keeper looking out from the safety of the lighthouse at the storm around us. We are separate from it. We can step out into the rain. We can get caught up in it. We can fight it. But we are not it.

When we step back from the emotion and see it as something separate, we begin to learn that we are able to manage it. We don't collapse. We are able to cope. It mightn't be perfect. It may even be very distressing, but it is nothing to be afraid of. It is the weather of our lives. No matter what the weather, we are able to manage it. When we stop catastrophising our own emotions, we learn that we are stronger than we thought; we may need some helpful behaviours but we are able to manage the weather whatever it may be.

POSITIVE BELIEFS ABOUT SELF

Often people with emotional dysregulation feel like fish out of water, therefore their self-esteem can be low. It's important then to be mindful of the fact that they are doing lots of positive things. They are doing lots of things that make them feel happier, make them feel less distressed. It is really important that they take credit for this. No one else is doing this work. If someone has adopted a new routine, has challenged their thoughts, has found some middle-way behaviour, has reduced how much they suppress, they deserve an enormous pat on the back. And it is no use this pat on the back coming from someone else. The person who needs to believe in them is them.

So take out the smartphone or laptop. For the next thirty days I would like you to try something. I would like you to write down every time you cope with something emotional: big things such as exams or meetings; small things such as infuriating siblings or frustrating colleagues. Begin to notice how well you are coping before you do a single thing. In fact, your whole life, you have been coping 90 per cent of the time. Sometimes it may have become too difficult and that's where we can add a few extra skills, but actually you have been managing every day for decades. It is just a fact. So it is important not to ignore it.

At the end of the month ask yourself: how often have I coped with negative emotions? How often have I managed, adapted, figured out, overcome, survived and handled negative emotions? Rather than seeing myself as someone who doesn't cope with emotion, perhaps I'm an expert navigator, someone who has dealt with extraordinary emotion that no one else would be able to manage.

So let's write it down. What have I done right in the past?

What am I doing right, at this moment in time?

What am I hoping to do right in the future?

What does this tell me about me? Maybe it tells me that emotion is part of my life but I am able to manage it. What does it say about me as a person? Maybe it tells me that I am stronger than I thought. Maybe it tells me that I am actually a very competent person. Maybe it tells me that sometimes my feelings get on top of me but actually I manage pretty well. I am able to surf the wave.

That doesn't mean that surfing the wave is easy. It can be tiring and difficult. Annoying bosses are annoying. There is no point pretending that they are not. So what can we do for ourselves? Let's make sure there are positive things for ourselves in every week. Regular kindnesses: appointments for a massage or facial. Then small, everyday kindnesses: splash out on that nice hand cream we like or treat ourselves to a cappuccino. Small kindnesses, just for us. Princess Diana said 'carry out a random act of kindness, with no expectation of reward, safe in the knowledge that one day someone might do the same for you'. I think she was wrong. I think this generates a level of expectation that other people will reciprocate our kindness. Often they won't or they won't do it when we actually need it. I think it creates a situation where we always put others first. Other people are important, but we are as important as anyone else. We can wait for other people to provide kindness but it is more important that we provide it ourselves. We have to recognise our own goodness, our own needs, our deservedness of love and kindness. There is something important in being kind to ourselves and not seeing this as something selfish, but vital. Something life-giving. Aesop, of 'The Hare and the Tortoise' fame, suggested: 'No act of kindness, no matter how small, is ever wasted.' This is true for others but it is also true for you. If other people are the only ones to provide kindness, then we are often the ones to provide criticism and cruelty that is not directed at others, but at ourselves. So we can adjust Princess Diana's quote to 'carry out a random act of kindness, once a day, just for you'. Then we'll start to recognise our own intrinsic worth.

INTERPERSONAL TRIGGERS

When you talk to people, the trigger for their distress is often very clear. The most common trigger is negative interpersonal interactions. Given that we Spaniards are used to not being understood by the Germans of the world, we are often very sensitive to potential rejections. We notice small slights. We misinterpret ambiguous comments. We can begin to worry very quickly about the things that people say and do. These negative interpersonal interactions are the most common trigger for our emotional dysregulation. Often the trigger for emotional dysregulation is the sense that we are being rejected by someone important in our lives. This rejection may be real or not, but the important thing is that we perceive it as real.

There are several things we can do. We can actually try to solve the problem with the other person. Often people with emotional dysregulation difficulties will duck, avoid, placate, do anything but actually solve the problem. Therefore it comes up again and again. If it is our boss, we can have a meeting and try to fix it. If it is our parent or our partner, we can try to talk to them about it. All the techniques around problem-solving (from the chapter 'Don't Worry Be Happy') should be useful here.

Some problems can't be solved. Maybe our neighbour is just a pain in the neck. We can try to organise things the best way we can but they may not see the world the way we see it. Sometimes then, we have to change our expectations of how people are going to be with us. Some neighbours are noisy. Some parents are controlling. Some siblings are infuriating. If we have unrealistic expectations about the nature of our relationships, then we are always likely to be disappointed. This disappointment is enough to trigger frustration, annoyance and other negative emotions. Sometimes we become angry at them; sometimes we become angry at ourselves.

We can feel that we have failed these people, that we should be better or different. The thoughts and expectations that these people generate in us often leads to our being critical of ourselves.

We can partake in extreme behaviour as we try to placate a boss or parent who will never change. Maybe we don't have to stand on our heads. Maybe we don't have to believe it is us who has the problem. Maybe it is not our fault they are the way they are. Maybe we don't have to change, but our expectations might. We mightn't be able to expect that they will like us, be nice to us, understand us, appreciate us, recognise our good points all the time. Maybe we have to be realistic about how people are. Abraham Lincoln hit the nail on the head when he said 'you can't please all of the people, all of the time'. Sometimes we have to accept that people are as they are. Good, bad, understanding, not understanding, and that sometimes those people are not going to be easy for us to get along with.

The first thing we did on this earth, as tiny embodiments of emotions and distress, was cry. The next thing we knew we were being comforted by the warmth of a blanket and the love of a mother. In our adult lives, we don't have a mother who will pick us up and comfort us. So when we are dealing with difficult people, we have to learn how to comfort ourselves. We have to learn how to be gentle and compassionate with ourselves. When is the time for the long bath, the hair cut, the massage, the football match on TV? We need to bring that compassion at the right time, and often that right time is just before or after having to deal with the difficult people in our lives.

CONCLUSION

It can be difficult being Spanish. We can feel things more than other people. Everything that seems natural to us is alien to people around us. They can be critical and judgmental because of it. We can feel overwhelmed with emotion and distress. We will never stop being who we are, but we don't have to feel as distressed as we sometimes do. We need to navigate ourselves towards the middle way, towards balanced behaviour and balanced thoughts, towards self-compassion and gentleness, towards self-kindness. This kindness calms the storm and allows us to be happy in our own knowledge of who we are.

How to Build a Happier Country

Mental Health and the Economy

The financial crisis and the housing bust created an environment in which everyone was trying to spend less, but my spending is your income and your spending is my income, so when everyone tries to cut spending at the same time the result is an overall decline in incomes and a depressed economy.

NOBEL LAUREATE IN ECONOMICS, PAUL KRUGMAN, 2014

Often when we talk about mental health, we talk about what is inside the person, and, of course, what is inside the person matters. But there is also a larger context. We are not separate from our environment, our economy, our society. In April 2014, the Irish parliament published a report highlighting how the financial crisis and subsequent recession were inextricably linked with the increase in suicides in Ireland over the previous five years. To those of us in the field of mental health, this was recognition of what we had been seeing day-to-day; it was merely stating the obvious. The stress of unemployment, reduced job security and increased financial pressure had significantly affected the well-being of vast swathes of society.

Although the relationship between mental health difficulties and financial hardship seems obvious, the human toll of the financial crisis is only beginning to be realised. This isn't a crisis that occurred in 2008. This is a crisis that started in 2008 and one that has the potential to run into the next decade. To really see the impact of the financial crisis on our well-being, we need to look at two things: (i) the psychological effects of a recession and (ii) the impact mental health problems have on the broader economy.

Let's come back to Richard Layard. He's an economist who has spent most of his adult life highlighting the importance of mental health both to the health of the nation and the health of a nation's economy. In his role as Programme Director of the Centre for Economic Performance in the London School of Economics, he has compiled a vast body of data showing how much mental health dominates issues of general health, unemployment, the justice system and personal happiness. Layard is very vocal on this issue. He believes the single biggest cause of unhappiness in our community arises from mental health difficulties. Not poverty, not crime, not physical health.

If we try to predict who is unhappy, we find that the strongest predictor is a person's prior mental illness. Prior mental illness explains more current unhappiness than poverty does.

Richard Layard[5]

Yet when he looked at services in the UK, he found that most of this illness goes untreated. In national surveys, only a quarter of those diagnosed were in treatment. Most of those in treatment were on medication prescribed by a GP, although the majority of patients would have preferred therapy. Even among those in a depressive episode, less than half were in treatment; only 8 per cent had seen a psychiatrist in the previous twelve months; and only 3 per cent had seen a psychologist.

THE PSYCHOLOGICAL EFFECTS OF RECESSION
The recession has put a huge financial burden on almost every home in Ireland. In 2012, 14.7 per cent of Irish people were unemployed. The ESRI Central Statistics Office estimates there

has been, on average, a 3 per cent drop in wages since 2008,[6] despite an increase in living costs. Taxes have been increased and those who are employed feel less secure in their jobs, have less take-home pay and are saddled with large mortgages. Large numbers of people have emigrated. People who are retired have seen their pensions reduced. People out of employment have been hit hardest of all. In the words of Shakespeare, 'all are punished'.

On an economic level, the effects of this are very clear. On a psychological level, people are under constant pressure due to a lack of money. Generally, one bad event doesn't make us psychologically unwell. It is the unrelenting repetition of negative events that does the damage. Whether we are unemployed or under financial stress, it is the continual pressure that affects us. The activities that would normally operate as stress relief, such as holidays and nights out, gradually get chopped back. Every month, it becomes a little bit harder and optimism becomes a little more dulled. It becomes a daily grind, as the individual and family have to curtail expenditure. Many choices parents have to make will also impact their children. Freedom and choice become eroded. It is very hard to see your children going without and not to feel that you are to blame. Newspapers talk of macroeconomic trends but in an average household this translates into money for school trips or sports clubs. Things we want to give but can't. Economic recession is theoretical; not having money is personal.

Freud spoke about the need for love and work. Financial pressure impacts upon both. When talking to people who are in financial difficulties it is surprising to find that often it is not work they focus on but love. They feel that they aren't fulfilling their role as parents if they can't provide what their children want. If they struggle to pay debts or make mortgage payments, they feel that they aren't fulfilling their role as a partner. They love the people around them and feel that they are failing them if they cannot provide them with the things that they need. Generally, people are actually providing an awful lot, but they feel they aren't returning their family's love and that can be devastating.

Financial constriction has a powerful affect on relationships: with our partners, our children and ourselves. It interferes with our marriages. We like to think that our relationships are beyond all that, but the reality is different. Our relationships are delicate things. Issues like stress and financial pressure have an impact on them. People under stress differ in what they prioritise, in how they cope, in the demands they make on each other. People under financial pressure are faced with life-changing choices: emigration, moving house, moving city. There is huge stress involved in making these decisions at the best of times. When we have to make them under financial pressure, the stress can be overwhelming. When we know that this is not the choice that we want to make, having to decide can make us feel helpless.

Decision fatigue is an important concept to understand here. Decisions that are easy to make at the beginning of the day become impossible by the end of the day, simply because of the amount of processing the brain has had to do to accommodate them. Over the last five years, Irish families have had to make decision after decision, and this process simply wears them down. They are often on their own, trying to figure out the best thing to do in impossible situations. They have to make decisions continually: huge ones about banks and loans and debts, and small ones about day-to-day necessities. This is true for families but it is also true in the workplace. A third of Irish businesses are small or medium enterprises (SMEs). For many people in SMEs there is no other person to run those decisions by. The Irish economy is perhaps unique in the number of people who work in family-run businesses: shops, SMEs, farms. Business decisions are family decisions and family decisions are business decisions. This increases the pressure when things start to go wrong. If a business has been in the family for a couple of generations, it increases the sense of loss if it closes. As people have to work through each decision, even positive events can seem negative, as people try to figure how they are going to manage.

UNEMPLOYMENT AND DEPRESSION

It is no surprise then that unemployment and mental health difficulties are related. Other than relationship difficulties, unemployment is the factor most likely to trigger depression. If we know that unemployment figures have spiked, then we know that the number of people suffering from depression will also have spiked. For over thirty years, we have seen research that describes a gradual increase in anxiety and depression, and a gradual decrease in confidence as the period of unemployment lengthens.

Despite a global financial crisis and a national recession, people still feel individually to blame if they lose their job. One of the consistent themes of therapy is the blame and self-criticism that come with reduced financial status. I have seen people worth a million euro and others worth a hundred euro coming to me with the same worries: '*what is my family going to think?*'; '*what are my friends going to think?*'; '*what am I if I am not the provider?*'; '*have I failed?*'

It is easy to identify the emotions that go with being unemployed. People feel low. They feel ashamed. People don't walk into a party and say that they are unemployed. There is a sense of stigma. It is something that people keep hidden. How many positive news stories are there about people who are unemployed? People feel it is their own doing and that they are somehow responsible. Psychologically, it is deeply personal. In the first few months after becoming unemployed, people can keep themselves busy. They can focus on home improvement, gardening or other projects, but this can quickly become unsatisfying. The inability to fill one's time meaningfully can lead to apathy and low motivation; once this happens, it becomes a vicious cycle: the less you do, the less you feel like doing.

The psychologist Marie Jahoda[7] identified five categories vital to well-being. They are:
1. Time structure
2. Social contact
3. Purpose
4. Social identity
5. Regular activity

We can see that employment will often address each of these categories, if not completely at least in a substantive way. We have a reason to get out of bed; we have a structure to the day; many jobs involve significant social contact with colleagues and clients; we have a role and responsibility. Work can give us a sense of identity. How many conversations start with someone enquiring as to what you do? How many conversations with friends and family start with 'how's work?' We can see that if we become unemployed each of Jahoda's categories would be significantly undermined. The basic structure of our day could be eroded. Our basic level of social contact and activity would plummet. Instead of meeting twenty people a day we might meet two. Our role and social identity are challenged. What happens when that sense of purpose disappears?

HOW CAN WE MANAGE THE RECESSION PSYCHOLOGICALLY?

Recessions are not easy psychologically. It is systemic. It is a problem individuals didn't create and it is often a problem individuals can't solve. No one individual can shift an economy. We just have to figure out how to manage and get ourselves through it. I hope that the previous chapters are useful in doing this. Each one is relevant in some way.

Jahoda's five categories are a good place to start. If we have lost our job, or had a significant change in circumstances, or are under significant stress we know that these categories are going to be challenged. Yet, psychologically, we need them. In work, out of work, under pressure, free of pressure, we need to ensure we have these categories covered in order to function. So we need to examine how to approach each category, no matter what our circumstances.

‣ **Regular activity:** we still need all the things we have always needed. To be out of the house. To be exercising. To spend time outdoors. To keep the brain active. It isn't always easy to work out how to do these things when our circumstances change, but it's important we make space for them.

‣ **Time structure:** we need to start looking at how our week is structured. What's my plan for getting up, going to bed? How is my day going to be structured?

‣ **Social contact:** there are few of us who do not need to see people: friends, neighbours, family. People who mean something to us or who give us a lift. Generally, when we are under pressure, we pull back from social contact. We need to move the other way. Who can we text/Skype/ have a cup of tea with/go for a walk with?

‣ **Purpose:** our job often gives us a sense of purpose. If that is jeopardised, we need to start looking at some of the other options that might help fulfil that need: volunteering; part-time work; unpaid work; helping out friends, neighbours or family members. Something we find meaningful. It doesn't have to be forever but it does have to be now.

‣ **Social identity:** when our circumstances change, we often disappear from our regular social circle. We feel ashamed, so we pull away. No one else thinks you are your job. They actually like you for you. Butcher, baker, candlestick-maker. Other people care much less about your job than you do.

As you read through the list above, I suspect lots of thoughts will rise to the surface if you have found yourself recently unemployed. I also suspect various emotions may have been triggered: anger and frustration at having to work on lists like this one; sadness at the loss of the way life had been; embarrassment at having to meet people; worry that life mightn't change. These are all the negative thoughts and feelings that hit people when their circumstances change.

Some of the most typical thoughts are:

'I am not fulfilling my role as a parent'
'I am not fulfilling my role as a partner'
'I am failing my family'
'What is my family going to think?'
'What are my friends going to think?'
'What am I, if I am not the provider?'
'Have I failed?'

As in the chapter on anxiety, let's see the above as Theory A, one way of understanding all the things that have happened. Theory A beliefs often push us into negative, anxious or embarrassed emotions, and escape or avoidant behaviours. If this constitutes Theory A, what would Theory B involve?

'I didn't create the recession, I am just doing my best to get through it.'
'I made some mistakes but so did Alan Greenspan, Tony Blair, Bertie Ahern and all the rest.'
'I have failed nobody. I love my family and ultimately that is all they need.'
'It is a pity that I can't give the kids the things they want, but

*nobody ever died from not having stuff. This generation still has
so much more than we did growing up.'*
'*I am not a provider. I'm a person. I work hard. I do my best and
that is all that can be expected of me.'*

See how different Theory B is. It is realistic. It is not saying
things are easy, but it is not laying the blame at your door or
saying that you have magic powers to fix it. It sees you as a
human being – not a job, a role or a provider.

Money matters. Life is stressful without it. But it is not who
you are. Sometimes we need to take a longer view. What will
all this look like from the vantage point of old age? The answer:
an unpleasant period of your life, but one that you survived.
Something you coped with and if you can cope with this you
can cope with anything.

THE IMPACT OF MENTAL HEALTH DIFFICULTIES ON THE ECONOMY

The London School of Economics has undertaken meticulous
work in highlighting that mental health isn't a niche subject. It
is relevant to every family, every community and can affect any
individual. Mental health accounts for a quarter of the global
burden of disease.

As mentioned earlier, the Department of Health has estimated
that the total economic cost of mental health problems in
Ireland is around €11 billion euro per year. The cost of providing
healthcare is only a small fraction of this. The majority of
the costs are due to the impact on the jobs market of lost
employment, absenteeism, reduced productivity and premature
retirement.[8] It is important to realise first how expensive mental
health problems are to the economy. Second, we could double
the budget for mental health treatment and it would still be the
smallest part of the cost of mental health difficulties. Third, any

improvement in people's mental health due to treatment is likely to pay dividends through reduced sick leave, reduced disability payment and increased productivity.

Across most western countries, less than half of people with mental health problems will receive treatment.[9] Mostly this will involve being prescribed medication, but only a tiny fraction will receive psychological treatment. There is no reason to think that Ireland's record of treating mental health difficulties is any better.

We know that one hundred and ten thousand people in Ireland receive disability benefit as a result of mental health difficulties, and this constitutes 33 per cent of all disability payments.[10] This has been steadily increasing over the last twenty years. When the World Health Organisation (WHO) looked at Ireland, it estimated that 29.6 per cent of the burden of disease was due to mental health difficulties.[11]

The My World Survey (2012) assessed six thousand secondary children. From that survey, we know that in Ireland right now, 40 per cent of young adults have elevated levels of anxiety and depression. Some of those children and young adults will manage and others won't. Which of those children will still be struggling with those mental health difficulties in twenty years' time?

In Ireland, as in other countries, mental health is the Cinderella of Government Departments. We only spend 6 per cent of our health budget on mental health related issues, despite its being an area of huge personal suffering and economic hardship. We spend the majority of this on hospital beds and on severe mental health difficulties, rather than on the most common mental health difficulties. We focus on reactive treatments when someone is already at crisis point, rather than early intervention or preventative treatment.

People may ask why mental health costs so much. There are two simple reasons. First, mental health difficulties are common. One in three people will experience a mental health problem in their lifetime and at any one point in time, one in six people will be experiencing a mental health difficulty. Second, mental health difficulties significantly interfere with our ability to live our day-to-day lives, to go to school or college or work and this comes at a cost. The first rule to understand is that if it is bad for our health, it is bad for our economy. If we drop out of college, lose a job, take sick leave or need employment support, it has a massive impact on the individual but it also has a huge impact on the wider economy. This means it is not just the individual's problem to deal with.

There is a complete disconnect between the gravity of mental health as a social issue and the societal response. Governments fell over the banking bailout. Governments barely discuss mental health. Even for those who don't see mental health as relevant to them, they can surely see how relevant its economic impact is. There is a huge disparity between the scale of the problem and current resources there to meet it. Thirty-three per cent of disability in Ireland is caused by mental health difficulties, but only 6 per cent of the health budget is allocated towards mental health. A sticking plaster. And that is all it can do. Services can be reorganised. Staff can work harder or better or smarter but it is David fighting Goliath, and realistically Goliath will win every time.

It is very common to think of mental health as an obscure issue. We used to think that if you didn't need to go to a psychiatric hospital there was no mental health difficulty. We now know that mental health affects large numbers of people; when something like the financial crisis hits, this is going to be reflected in the number of people experiencing mental health difficulties. If there is a financial crisis, then there is going to be a mental health crisis not far behind. We have been talking about unemployment leading to depression, but of course it also goes in the other direction. The longer someone is depressed, the harder they find it to get back to work. This can cause lifelong unemployment. Initially this is an economic problem causing a mental health problem, but relatively quickly it becomes a mental health problem causing an economic problem.

Everyone knows it is hard to get back to work even if an economy starts to improve. There are months of searching the employment pages; rethinking what you might do and how you might fit in a new jobs market; filling out the applications; receiving the rejections; attending the interviews. We know how interviews work: see six people to fill one post. This means we are likely to have to do six interviews to get one job. All of this takes motivation, drive, energy and optimism; all the qualities that can be eroded by mental health difficulties. As well as being able to cope with the practicalities of a job search, people have to be ready to work on their mental health in order to deal with the attendant challenges and potential rejections.

Stress, pressure and challenges to our self-esteem – these are all associated with just looking for work. They are all factors that lead to mental health difficulties, and the longer we have been depressed the harder it is for us to challenge them and return to the workforce. Economic growth or recession won't matter. Someone's health will be the primary difficulty standing in their way of returning to work. We often think of the human cost of a crisis as separate from the financial cost, but the two go hand in hand.

Will the new role be in an area the applicant has experience in? Will a fifty-year-old with years of experience in the construction industry be suitable for an entry-level job in the service industry? Our concept of who we are is very connected to what we do. What happens when there is a disconnect between how we see ourselves and the available jobs? If I previously earned fifty thousand euro a year sitting at a desk, what happens to my self-esteem when the jobs available offer a salary that's only half that amount and involve standing on my feet?

The idea that all we need to do to get people back to work is to create jobs sadly misses all the evidence from previous recessions.

When we look at the 1980s in Ireland, or the closing of the mines in Wales, or the closing of heavy industry in Northern England, we see that unemployment can quickly become generational and that this is only partly due the economic context at the time. The Government needs to tackle the connection between unemployment and depression now before Ireland has a chronic mental health/unemployment deadlock throughout the next decade.

Those with mental health problems who are unemployed are doubly stigmatised. Despite the prevalence of mental health difficulties and the fact that complete recovery is the most common outcome, mental health problems are second only to HIV/AIDS in terms of the level of stigma. The WHO believes that stigma is one of the greatest challenges to recovery facing people with mental health difficulties. Stigma is endemic across all aspects of the employment process.

‣ People with mental health problems find it more difficult to obtain work; about half of employers do not wish to employ a person with a psychiatric diagnosis. Yet, in reality only 15 per cent of employers who employ people with mental health difficulties report it as having been a negative experience.

‣ People with mental health problems are more likely to be underemployed or in poorly paid jobs.

‣ People with mental health problems frequently report being denied opportunities for training, promotion or transfer.

‣ People with mental health problems know about stigma. They worry about being judged. Many people go to great lengths to prevent colleagues knowing they have been ill. This attempt at concealment can make people reluctant to request time off for doctor's appointments or therapy sessions. It reduces their chance of obtaining appropriate support from occupational health or employee assistance programmes. Ultimately stigma can stop us getting well or keeping a job.

In its recent report, the OECD gave this advise to all modern economies:

> If labour markets are to function well, it is important that policy makers address the interplay between mental health and work. They are slowly coming to recognise that they have long neglected an issue that is critical to people's well-being and for contributing to sustainable economic growth. The policy changes required are substantial and involve a large number of institutions and stakeholders working towards better co-ordinated policies and service delivery. Reform will therefore require strong political leadership. The consolidated set of social, education, health, and labour market policy responses that are needed to promote better mental health and employment outcomes are the focus of this report.
>
> OECD[12]

Economic researchers in University College Galway looked at the economic arguments for increasing spending on mental health in Ireland. They could find no economic underpinning for the ongoing *low* level of spending. They found economic evidence for a series of interventions. They suggested a target of increasing mental health spending to 10 per cent of the health budget over a five-year period; a greater integration between community services and specialist services; greater support to return to work; and societal level interventions to reduce stigma. They even found evidence that people would be willing, if necessary, to pay more tax to achieve this.

This was the summary of their advise to the Irish Government:

> Our research in the following chapters can be summarised as follows: policy makers cannot afford

> *not* to invest in mental health; service providers
> and researchers in Ireland need better data for any
> extra investment to yield the maximum returns
> for individuals, society and the economy; advocacy
> groups and researchers need to increase their efforts
> to persuade the public that increased investment in
> mental health services represents a wise and just use of
> resources.
>
> O'Shea and Kennelly 2006 (their emphasis)

So if improved mental health care is in everyone's best interest, why have we not made the right changes to our policies and supports? There are probably a number of reasons. It is only in very recent years that advocates have broken through the silence that has surrounded mental health. We have only started to be able to talk about mental health at a policy level and not just as a personal 'tragedy'. There has been a huge benefit in celebrities, sports stars and others coming forward to discuss their experiences. It has humanised an issue that was hidden away, and as soon as we see the people behind the issue then we can start working to address it.

Our general ignorance of mental health has created therapeutic hopelessness among policy makers. This is simply not the therapeutic reality.

There is a wide range of highly cost-effective treatments that are short, intensive and effective. If you are interested in what these are go to nice.org.uk. NICE is the National Institute of Clinical Excellence. It is a non-governmental, non-pharmaceutical organisation that collects all the published evidence in any area of medicine. It compares all the trials and states what has the best evidence based on those findings. Often NICE is only in the news when it says a new drug isn't as good as the pharmaceutical company has suggested that it is. It publishes evidence-based treatments for every different mental health problem on its website. It is free and there are user-friendly versions as well as the versions with all the statistics.[13]

What will it tell you? There are numerous options – prevention strategies, early intervention services, low-intensity treatments, psychological treatments, community-based interventions – that could improve the lives of people in Ireland if only they had access to them. These are all evidence-based, pragmatic interventions that will save lives in our localities and ultimately billions of euro for the Department of Finance. The outcomes for every mental health disorder have the potential to be far better than they currently are. We don't have to invent anything. We just have to provide the treatments that are already there and that other countries have access to.

What exists? Effective psychological treatments for:
‣ Eating disorders
‣ Self-harm
‣ Depression
‣ Post-Traumatic Stress Disorder
‣ Social anxiety
‣ Health anxiety
‣ Obsessive Compulsive Disorder
‣ Panic attacks
‣ Psychoses such as schizophrenia

The average cost of a psychological intervention for the first two disorders is €2,400. For all the other disorders it is €1,200. These are difficult to access in Ireland. All of them work for the majority of people who use them. All of them would lead to social and economic benefit to Irish society. Consider how cheap treatments are when compared to the cost of long-term unemployment or disability to the exchequer. The London School of Economics suggests that if even 5 per cent of people who received psychological interventions returned to the workforce, it would pay for the treatment of the other 95 per cent. People often suggest that treatment is expensive; however, it's not half as expensive as a lack of treatment.

Yet in practice, it feels that mental health is never supported in a way that could meet the scale of the challenge. In order to do this, any Irish Government has to focus on:

‣ **prioritisation of mental health services:** not allowing physical health overruns to eat into the development of mental health services

‣ **outcome-based treatments:** not just funding the same old services but reinforcing services that lead to lasting improvements in people's well-being, including an extra emphasis on psychological and social treatments

‣ **implementation:** any new service needs national roll-out so that some catchments don't thrive while others struggle.

These are all interventions that have little or no focus on capital expenditure. They are dependent on a flexible, well-trained work force. In this respect, they are relatively easy to roll out nationally and open to adapting and changing in the future as needs be.

Mental Health and Irish Society

We discovered two astonishing things about the rate of depression across the century. The first was there is now between ten and twenty times as much of it as there was fifty years ago. And the second is that it has become a young person's problem. When I first started working in depression thirty years ago ... the average age of which the first onset of depression occurred was 29.5 ... Now the average age is between fourteen and fifteen.

MARTIN SELIGMAN

The subject of mental health is a highly contentious one. It involves issues to do with removing people's liberty; the rise of the use of psychiatric medication among adults and children; labels and stigma; the medicalisation of human emotion; vast billions of euro in disability payments and lost earnings; and overwhelming human suffering. These issues are highly controversial, highly costly, and go to the core of what it means to be human. Mental health is an important part of society.

In 2010, the World Health Organisation[14] looked at all the causes of death and disease across the world to assess their impact. They looked at data from one hundred and eighty-seven countries. When they looked at all diseases (including AIDS, malaria, malnutrition and war), mental health disorders and substance use disorders were the fifth leading cause of death and disease worldwide. They accounted for 23 per cent of the total global burden of disease. Depressive disorders were the most common mental health difficulty, followed by anxiety disorders and drug use disorders. The highest level of social disability occurred in people aged ten to twenty-nine years of age. This was true across all western countries. In most cases, suicide, rather than any physical ailment, was the highest cause of mortality in men under thirty.

These findings are vital to understanding that mental health and mental health services are not remote or minority public policy issues. Mental health is a significant component of society. It is the elephant in the room of public policy; it is so significant we have to start talking about it.

Such findings are important because they tell us that we are not alone. Even if we feel we are the only person experiencing a mental health problem, it is vital that we know this is common, it is not our fault and it is occurring throughout society. It is also vital that we know how *normal* it is. Mental health disorders are common and they are primarily diseases of the young.

Why is this happening? Life has improved immeasurably in Ireland over the last thirty years. We live longer, eat better, go on holidays more frequently. Many of us have opportunities in terms of work, relationships and leisure activities that would have been unimaginable just a few decades ago. Yet even for those of us not experiencing a mental health difficulty, it seems like we are more stressed than ever before. What's going on? Well, we have had a financial crisis but that doesn't explain everything. In fact, people were becoming stressed and unwell before the crisis and, even when it is resolved, it is likely that we will continue to have difficulties. This chapter is in no way a complete review of the stresses in society, but it gives a snapshot of some of the major difficulties we all face.

WOMEN

Most women have greater freedom than their mothers or grandmothers. Women can vote, work, go to college and marry whom they choose. Dublin has recently named one of the major bridges across the River Liffey after Rosie Hackett, an early pioneer of feminism in Ireland. If Rosie Hackett were alive today, she would see some remarkable changes. Yet, she would be hard pressed to say that there is equality. You would be hard pressed to say that the twenty-first century hasn't created a whole range of new pressures for women.

Women are still often paid less than their male counterparts. In terms of their career development, they still face a glass ceiling, and because they often take time out to have children and raise a family, their final pensions are often smaller. There are significantly fewer women in positions of power and influence than men. The care many women provide in the home for children and elderly or sick relatives is often undervalued, despite its significant financial and societal importance. Women remain primarily responsible for maintaining household budgets and running the family. They experience the threat of violence in their homes and on the street.

The most common stress that I see women experiencing in therapy results from the demands of these multiple roles. They would like to have a family and be a mother; they are also talented and well-educated and would like to maintain their career; they would like a relationship in which they feel loved and supported; while also maintaining their well-being and friendships. Yet in the modern world these understandable desires often end up competing with each other.

There appears to be a tacit belief in society that it's somehow possible for women to juggle all these responsibilities. There appears to be a societal expectation that women should be able to multitask all day, every day. No one ever seems to say that there is a personal cost to this: stress, exhaustion, feelings of guilt or failure.

A female employee can feel guilty for taking maternity leave and may feel under pressure to come back to work as soon as possible. When she does she may feel guilty about having to leave her child in crèche during the working week. If she leaves the office at five o'clock with work unfinished, she feels she is letting her employer or colleagues down; if she works late she feels she is letting her child down.

Flexitime, job-sharing and sabbaticals are all worthwhile initiatives when it comes to making life easier for working women, but all too often they are resisted by employers. There is no reason that the forty-hour week is the only way to organise society. Our structures are twentieth century but our lives are twenty-first century. We share responsibility. Money is important but it is not everything. We want to see our children.

I once worked in an organisation with fifty staff. I was the only one working nine to five, Monday to Friday. Everyone else worked part time. I found this bewildering at first. It transpired because most of the staff were female, the management had put in place policies to manage maternity leave and childcare twenty years earlier. They could have gone down an aggressive letter-of-the-law tack but instead took an enlightened approach and encouraged employees to work part time. The company had a staff retention rate that was second to none. They built a reservoir of expertise, knowledge and loyalty. Staff worked exceptionally hard on the days they were there and retained an enthusiasm for the work twenty and thirty years after starting.

Many women want to have children and a family, but if we presume that everyone has an easy time getting pregnant then we are not recognising a new reality in Irish society. With couples now getting married later in life, difficulties around childbirth have increased significantly. The average age of a groom in 1977 in Ireland was twenty-six. In 2015 it's thirty-five and women show a similar pattern. WHO data indicates that one in five couples in Ireland now have difficulties conceiving, which is the highest rate in Europe.

That getting pregnant can be hard, that pregnancy can be difficult and that childbirth can be physically and psychologically traumatic – these are issues that people don't talk about. There is a silence about the reality of how hard creating a new human being can be. If we fail to get pregnant then we can end up blaming ourselves for something we have no control over. It used to be common for women to die in childbirth. Thankfully, that seldom happens in Ireland now but it doesn't mean we should neglect how significant a physical event it is. One-fifth of all pregnancies end in miscarriage; labour can be deeply traumatic and can take people weeks or even months to recover from, both physically and emotionally. These are not small events, but societal expectations appear to have shifted to the extent that women are expected to bounce back to their former selves with little consideration of the challenging experience they have just had.

Women are under extraordinary pressure to do what can't be done: everything. There is a silent expectation on women to do it all, to the extent that if they choose to stay at home, that feels like a failure. If they don't have children, that feels like a failure. If they imperfectly balance the two, that feels like a failure. People often personalise the difficulties they are experiencing: '*I should be able to do whatever is asked of me.*' On the other hand, the demands of society never get identified as unrealistic. Someone is up five times in the night to feed a baby and it is their fault that they feel stressed in work the next day? Their stress isn't understood as a reasonable response. It is seen as a problem.

MEN

The twenty-first century has been interesting and difficult for men. In the past, although men were given great power in a predominantly patriarchal society, they were often denied full emotional relationships with their partners and children.

Something that we know is generally unhealthy, emotional suppression, was and is, seen as the core of 'manliness'. 'Real men' were stoic, stiff-upper-lipped, gruff males. Heroes were John Wayne and Clint Eastwood types – men who got the job done but didn't feel too much inside. Yet this denies an integral part of our humanity: whether we like it or not we are inherently emotional creatures.

Men will often come to therapy because they are troubled by what they feel but they also may be worried that they *feel* at all. They feel grief, feel loneliness, feel worry, feel unsure. These are emotions that you could not possibly go through life without encountering, regardless of gender. Yet they are seen as faults and weaknesses, something to be hidden. This wholly outdated perception has definitely improved, but no one would claim we have reached an age of emotional enlightenment. More recently, men are beginning to be placed in the same double bind that women have experienced for a much longer time. Men are struggling with many of the same difficulties that come up regularly for their partners and wives. They want to have a relationship with their children yet much of the societal perception of 'man as provider' is as strong as ever. There is still a demand to stay in the office late, to be on the road for several hours, to commute internationally if that is what the job demands. Concepts such as paternity leave are often ridiculed. Yet men need a balance in their lives and struggle to get it.

What happens to the 'man as provider' model when a recession hits? This core concept of what it is to be a man is undermined.

Research has shown that one in seven men who become unemployed will develop depression within the following six months. In 2014, the ESRI[15] showed that although everyone in Ireland had been impacted by the recession, men had been the most significantly hit. Researchers in the *British Journal of Psychiatry*[16] have dubbed the recent global economic downturn the 'mancession' for its singular impact on males in western economies. As myopic and controversial as such a title may be, there are several reasons to think that males might be at particular risk in the current slump. American researchers[17] suggest that 75 per cent of all the jobs lost in US since 2008 have men's. Although there have been major job losses across the economy, traditionally male industries such as construction and manufacturing have been hit particularly hard. In contrast, healthcare and education (which have a larger female workbase) have yet to see the same level of job losses.

Men are likely to experience several specific difficulties associated with mental health. If someone's identity is connected to their work, when they lose their job their world can fall apart. It is an experience that can shatter someone's self-esteem. A man's role within the family and within the community at large can feel diminished. It is not an exaggeration to say that often because men value work, if it is taken away then they value themselves less.

While isolation is in no way the preserve of men, as a general rule they have a smaller group of friends and rely on colleagues for social contact more so than women. Isolation is a key problem in depression as it reduces the social support that someone has access to and increases the room for negative thinking and worry. Men are less likely to talk, especially about emotion, and so can often struggle to manage the natural emotions that come with losing a job.

In all aspects of health, men are slower and less likely to seek help than women. This often means that men engage only in a crisis. While the experience of depression isn't radically different for men and women, one disparity stands out: the number of suicides. When looking at British data, the *British Medical Journal*[18] found that a 10 per cent increase in unemployed men led to a 1 per cent increase in suicide rates. Recent Irish data from the National Suicide Research Foundation suggested that close to five hundred cases of suicide were as a direct result of the economic crash. We need to look beyond the statistics and speak to the people experiencing depression. Recession is not merely an economic issue, it is a human one.

EQUAL RIGHTS

I live near the house that Oscar Wilde grew up in. Opposite is a statue of Oscar reclining. As he memorably put it, what he felt was 'the love that dare not speak its name'. Something intrinsic to who he was as a human being could not be spoken about. Albeit very recently, it feels like the world is opening up. People are celebrated in society in positions from where they would once have been fired. People can marry and be with the one they love in the eyes of the law and in society. The core of the gay experience, love, is being accepted.

Yet, there is still large-scale discrimination, violence, exclusion and a sense of gay people being 'other'. There are still higher rates of mental health difficulties among people who are gay often due to a sense of exclusion from the outside world and then an internal experiencing of self-stigmatising and not belonging.

This speaks to a larger issue of our ongoing taboo concerning sex. Sex appears to be everywhere but only in its most unrealistic forms. The presumption that everyone else's sex life is active, problem free and easy doesn't recognise the extraordinary complexity and variation throughout everyone's sex lives. Sex is everywhere, but the reality of what it is to be a sexual being is barely discussed. Sex is physically complicated. Sex is emotionally complex. Sexuality and attraction are amorphous. The freedom of the early gay rights movement and the conversations it started has a lot to teach broader society about being open in our discussions of sex and sexuality.

CHILDREN AND YOUNG PEOPLE

The experience of children has changed utterly over the course of the twentieth century. Key tenets of parenting – 'Children were to be seen and not heard'; 'Spare the rod and spoil the child' – are now seen as barbaric. Yet anyone over forty will recognise this was a core part of the philosophy that they grew up with. Corporal punishment was the norm. Children were taken, adopted, moved and abandoned.

A sorry and significant chapter of twentieth-century Irish history involves the emotional, physical and sexual abuse and neglect of children. I have recently worked with a significant number of men who were beaten regularly in school for being left-handed. What sort of insanity was that? And this wasn't back in Charles Dickens' time. This was considered modern Ireland.

Thankfully there have been many changes. Corporal punishment is now illegal and society understands that a child's emotional development is paramount. Children's rights are now enshrined in the constitution, but many of the scars of those experiences still exist. Many people still struggle with experiences that they never caused or could control. The legacy of how we treated children is all around us.

This is not to suggest that we are now living in some kind of utopia. Children feel the impact of poverty, a shortfall in social housing and dysfunction within the home most keenly. I don't think any of us believe that these issues have gone away.

There is something fundamental about mental health that we must recognise. It is primarily a disease of the young. You are most likely to develop mental health difficulties between the ages of fifteen and twenty-five. This is true in Ireland and internationally. We often regard difficulties like depression or anxiety as a middle-aged problem. They aren't. We often dismiss young people's difficulties with a flippant '*they'll grow out of it*', thus ignoring their potential seriousness.

The period between fifteen and twenty-five is one of enormous change as people leave the family home, begin to live independently and make decisions in relationships and careers. These are huge decisions and with them come huge pressures. Young people don't want to make mistakes. They try to balance safety with adventure, achievement with joyousness, independence with continuing closeness to those they know and love. This is a difficult balancing act and it is not surprising that they risk falling over.

We live in a superficial culture, where everyone is meant to be energised and positive all the time. Nowhere is this more keenly felt than among young people. They can feel that they are not living up to their potential or that they are less successful than their peers. They can feel that they don't have enough friends or that their experiences are lacking in some fundamental way. In a culture where achievement is lionised, ordinary day-to-day living can seem second rate.

Young people need money but don't have it. They need independence but struggle to achieve it. They need to balance the exceptionally competitive demands of college or the job market with a full and fulfilling social life. It is not easy and the statistics reflect this. The demands of living an 'adult' life are placed on the shoulders of younger and younger people who don't necessarily have the emotional skills to cope. Stress sets in when demands outweigh our capacity to deal with them. For young people, those demands come from all quarters.

GOOD NEWS

Well, that all sounds fairly grim. Except it's not that simple. There is a lot of good news. Eight out of ten people in Ireland regard themselves as happy. Seven out ten young people in Ireland regard themselves as happy. We have voted ourselves one of the happiest countries in the world. There have been steps towards positive change in every area of inequality. Yet the social stresses that cause mental health difficulties continue to be obvious.

There is a chronic need for an improvement in mental health services, but mental health is not just an issue for services to deal with. It is a community issue, and unless the larger community embraces and engages with mental health then it will always be destined to have poor outcomes. Any illnesses that society judges to be outside the 'norm' – be that male cancers, HIV or mental health problems – are destined to have a poor prognosis. It is only when society is willing to address these illnesses openly that real change can be made.

We need people to love, who love us in return, and an occupation that gives us a sense of meaning and satisfaction. But these are things that a mental health service cannot provide. It can keep us alive, help us get off the floor, it can allow us to see the world in a different light. But love, belonging and work, these come from our friends, family and from the whole community.

Loneliness kills. Research repeatedly reinforces that isolation drives and maintains every mental health disorder. Yet isolation cannot be addressed by a mental health service. It is incumbent on all of us to build the bonds of friendship and support that break through these feelings. One of the key findings[19] in recent research on young adults is that if a young person has one adult in their lives that they feel they can trust and talk to, this acts as a protective factor for all difficulties, and helps them overcome any problems they come across. I would solidly bet that the same applies to adults. If we can find one good friend, partner or support to help us through the difficult times, this will act as a powerful protective factor. The power of a cup of tea should never be underestimated.

We know that community initiatives are really helpful and that people really enjoy and respond positively to them. As stigma falls away and we talk about mental health more, we are able to support each other in ways that never happened before. Can we do anything to inoculate ourselves from modern life? No. Life will continue to be busy and complicated.

Yet the economic crisis may have given us a wonderful opportunity. As a community we have the chance to rethink some of our assumptions about the type of lives we want and the type of society we want to live in. We can look to emphasise happiness. We can look to emphasise community. Ireland recently won the The Good Country Index. This index suggests that per head of population Ireland does more for other people on the planet than any other country. It is something we can very proud of. It didn't happen by accident. It happened due to a long series of decisions and priorities that Irish society and especially the generation of the 1960s made. They prioritised peacekeeping, aid to developing countries, support of the arts. They looked to science and technology. That generation built an outward-looking modern nation.

At this moment in time, as a society, we are in a state of confusion. We can look to rebuild an economy or we can look to build a society. The things we prioritise now have the potential to define our country for a generation.

Psychologists have a strange perspective on society. We are immersed in others' unhappiness. We see the personal toll of broken relationships, traumas and unemployment. Yet, we often dream of remaking the world, to protect the people that we see from the suffering they face. We dream of a happier society. The more I read the less it seems like a dream. It seems achievable. There are many practical, concrete steps available to create it. A happier society can be built. Step by step. Decision by decision. Policy by evidence-based policy. The 1960s generation built a modern society. The post-crash generation can build a happier society.

There are a wide number of practical things we can do:
‣ We can recognise that most people, men and women, want a job and a family, and we have to make that balancing act easier.

We can legislate and incentivise job-sharing, part-time work opportunities, affordable childcare and improved maternity and paternity leave. These are achievable, practical policies that ensure work and life are not in constant competition. Nor are they anti-economic. There is strong evidence that they improve staff loyalty, staff retention and productivity.

› We can increase job security and ban zero-hour and low-hour contracts. Job insecurity is a recipe for stress and illness. High job satisfaction rates lead to lower absenteeism and higher productivity. This is an economic benefit to everyone. Work can't be a zero-sum game. It can be one of the most fulfilling aspects of our lives. But there is lots of evidence to suggest that the happier we are in our jobs, the harder we work. Legislation has to incentivise large employers to do the right thing. Paradoxically, employers will benefit in the long term. Short-term contracts, zero-hour contracts, and jobs without career paths mean we stop treating people as people but as automatons. We shouldn't be surprised then if people clock-watch, call in sick, are unproductive or unengaged. Happiness pays. The research says so.

› We can recognise that mental health is a normal part of health. If a company has two thousand employees, some will have cardiac problems or mobility issues, others mental health problems. Therefore, treatment, support and inclusion of staff with mental health difficulties is a necessity. We can no longer pretend mental health problems don't exist.

› We can increase knowledge, skills and training for employers in order to reduce work stress. This isn't about people working less hard, it is about realistic demands over a significant period of time, so that we maximise people's well-being and therefore their efficiency.

› We need nationwide stigma reduction campaigns. There needs to be a national acceptance of the normality of mental health difficulties, in schools, hospitals and large employers. If mental health problems are seen to damage careers then people hide them, problems escalate and only emerge following a crisis. This doesn't benefit anyone.

‣ Large-scale mental health awareness training for teachers, nurses, sports coaches, managers and anyone who interacts with large numbers of people.

‣ If communities want to protect their own, we need to reach out to those who are isolated and most vulnerable. We need to find ways to give a sense of self-worth to those who have lost their jobs or who are struggling. Because this could be any of us, at any stage. This is most effective coming from the community up. We can use the community structures already there, like gyms, churches and GAA clubs, to help target mental health difficulties through exercise, meditation, volunteering, etc. There is a large range of volunteer organisations which encourage us to re-engage with the world around us. There is also a whole raft of new social entrepreneur organisations to reach out to people who have become isolated and separated from their community. This isn't new. Neighbours always used to look after neighbours. This is what Ireland used to be like. We have just forgotten how to do it. The ordinary can be life-changing and the absence of the ordinary is devastating.

If someone does become unwell, mental illness does not have to be long term. Contradicting old stereotypes, the average length of depression, for instance, is eighteen months. That eighteen months is too long but it is not the lifelong suffering that many people picture when they think of mental health difficulties. For the majority of people, medication works. For the majority of people, psychological therapies work. Research tells us that self-help books, large-scale psychology workshops, computer-based therapy all work for different people at different points in their distress. Many of us are vulnerable to mental health problems but equally the vast, vast majority of us will get through it.

‣ Looking after the nation's mental health cannot be an accidental priority. A fundamental part of creating a happier society is helping reduce unhappiness. There are two key difficulties in terms of mental health service provision.

1. We need to develop better treatments. Treatments that have better outcomes so that we are able to help people in all their complexity. There is a range of conditions that need better interventions than we currently have the knowledge to address effectively. This means research funding into outcome-based treatment needs to be prioritised.

2. We need better access to the treatments that already exist. Too many people go too long without any input, and too many people go too long with access to only medication, without any psychological therapy.

‣ There is a huge range of effective treatments that could be provided
   - Home treatment
   - Early intervention treatments for vulnerable young people
   - Services focused on fifteen- to twenty-five-year-olds
   - Mental Health A+E
   - Drop-in services and long-term support
   - Access to psychological therapy via the internet
   - Access to psychological therapy via community groups
   - Access to psychological therapy via GP services and primary care services
   - Access to specialist CBT for anxiety disorders and depression
   - Greater access to physical and psychological treatments for eating disorders
   - Dialectical Behaviour Therapy – therapy to help people change patterns of behaviour that are harmful – for Borderline Personality Disorder
   - We need to integrate charity and voluntary groups to ensure national coverage and reduce crossover.

- We need to integrate public health, primary care services and crisis care on an organisational and service level.

All of these are cheaper and more effective than classical service models. There are hundreds of other policies that could be examined. They are neither policies of the left or the right. They are not owned by any party or group. They are not pro-business or anti-business. When you look at changes that are focused on the individual, and place the person's well-being at their core, it brings economic benefit with it. The things that harness our strengths and protect our vulnerabilities as individuals help build a stronger economy and a happier society.

When you think of Irish society, you can only be filled with hope. A nation carved out of history by sheer willpower. Generations who built lives and raised families through poverty. A sense of community hardwired into the Irish psyche. Optimism, humour and joyousness as national characteristics. If we choose to create a happier society, we can do it. One decision at time. One policy at a time. The impact felt by one person at a time.

HOPE

There are a lot of reasons to be hopeful. The evidence here and abroad appears to be clearer and clearer. It is in everyone's best interest to provide better mental health care. The WHO, OECD, LSE and every Department of Health think so. This isn't about justice or fairness or kindness. Our own self-interest is enough. Better mental health care pays for itself in reduced costs to the larger economy. Mental health care isn't charity. It's common sense. There is nothing more expensive that doing things badly. The cost of treatment is a tiny fraction of the cost of illness. I'm hopeful because I believe that common sense will prevail. On a purely economic level, better care is cheaper. So let's provide better care.

The other reason I am filled with hope is far away from complex economic data. I'm hopeful because, for the first time in history, we have a range of interventions that work and we have a community that is determined to provide them for people: through books, workshops, websites, apps, support groups, occupational groups, meditation groups, therapists and services. People are receiving care and support who never would have before.

The final reason I'm hopeful is that every day thousands of people recover from mental health difficulties and go on to be the wonderful, unique individuals they always were. The light sometimes flickers but is never extinguished. The extraordinary resilience of the human person is an ongoing inspiration. In meeting those people every day, my hope is constantly renewed.

Endnotes

1. Moorey, S. (2010), 'The six cycles maintenance model: growing a vicious flower for depression', *Behavioural and Cognitive Psychotherapy*, 38, 2, 173–184.

2. Layard, R. (2006), *The Depression Report: A New Deal for Depression and Anxiety Disorders*, London: London School of Economics.

3. Salkovskis, P. M. (1991), 'The importance of behaviour in the maintenance of anxiety and panic; a cognitive account', *Behavioural and Cognitive Psychotherapy*, 19, 1, 6–19.

4. Wells, A. (1997), *Cognitive Therapy for Anxiety Disorders*, Sussex: Wiley.

5. Layard, R. (2006), *The Depression Report*, London School of Economics: London.

6. Central Statistics Office (2015), Earning and Labour Costs Annual Report.

7. Jahoda, M. (1980), *Work, employment and unemployment: an overview of ideas and research results in the social science literature*, Sussex: University of Sussex Press.

8. O'Shea, E. & Kennelly, B. (2008), *The Economics of Mental Health Care in Ireland*, Mental Health Commission.

9. Brugha. T. et al. (2004), 'Trends in service use and treatment for mental disorders in adults throughout Great Britain', *British Journal of Psychiatry*, 185(5), 378–384.

10. National Disability Survey Ireland (2008), Cork: Central Statistics Office.

11. Whiteford et al. (2013), 'Global Burden of disease attributable to mental and substance use disorders: findings from the Global Burden of Disease Study 2010', *The Lancet*, 382, 9904, 1575–1586.

12. The OECD Mental Health and Work Policy Framework (2015), The Hague, OECD.

13. Layard and Clarke discuss how you can apply the best research based treatments to a whole society in their book *Thrive*.

14. Whiteford et al. (2013), 'Global Burden of disease attributable to mental and substance use disorders: findings from the Global Burden of Disease Study 2010', *The Lancet*, 382, 9904, 1575–1586.

15. McGinty, F., et al. (2014), *Winners and Losers: The Equality Impact of the Great Recession in Ireland*, Dublin: ESRI

16. Dunlop, B. & Mletzko, T. (2011), 'Will current economic trends produce a depressing future for men?' *British Journal of Psychiatry*, 198(3), 167–168.

17. Taylor et al. (2010), *Women and the New Economics of Marriage*, Pew Research Centre.

18. Barr, B. et al. (2012), 'Suicides associated with the 2008-2010 economic recession in England' *British Medical Journal*, 345: e5142.

19. Dooley, B. Fitzgerald, A. (2012), My World Survey, Dublin: Headstrong.